Prime-Time Style

Prime-Time Style

The Ultimate TV Guide to Fashion Hits— and Misses

Valerie Frankel
and
Ellen Tien

A PERIGEE BOOK

A Perigee Book
Published by The Berkley Publishing Group
200 Madison Avenue
New York, NY 10016

Copyright ©1996 by Ellen Tien and Valerie Frankel
Book design by H Roberts Design
Cover design by Joe Lanni
Front-cover photograph of Heather Locklear from The Kobal Collection; all other front-cover photographs from Movie Star News.

First edition: December 1996

Published simultaneously in Canada.

The Putnam Berkley World Wide Web site address is
http://www.berkley.com/berkley

Library of Congress Cataloging-in-Publication Data
Frankel, Valerie.
    Prime-time style: the ultimate TV guide to fashion hits—and misses/Valerie Frankel
and Ellen Tien. —1st ed.
        p. cm
    "A Perigee book."
    ISBN 0-399-52261-1
    1. Television programs—United States—Plots, themes, etc. 2. Costume.
I. Tien, Ellen. II. Title.
PN1992.3.U5F68 1996
791.45'75—dc20   96-36378
                                                        CIP

Printed in the United States of America

10 9 8 7 6 5 4 3 2 1

To Glenn and Will

Contents

Acknowledgments

Thanks to Julia, Chi, and Anita Tien, Judy, Howie, Alison Frankel, and Maggie Rosenberg for always understanding; Suzanne Bober for coming up with the whole idea and having the rare ability not to panic when everyone else did; Julie Merberg for assuring us that it would all be worth it one of these days; Stefanie Antoine for filling in the gaps; Caroline Hwang for serving above and beyond the call of duty; Carole Frazier and Shirley Wachter of the Costume Designers Guild for being the ultimate sources; Steven Berg, Kim Lepine, Grant McCracken, and Rick Marin for their expert opinions; Bunny Betts, Max and Lee Rosenberg, and Debbie Timothy for making life a little more comfortable; Frank Rosenberg for the motivation; John Boyer for his continuing pattern of perfection; and finally, Marshall "The Cage" Sella for top editing—come hell or accidental water—and tirelessly helping us keep the com in sitcom.

And special thanks to the costume designers who provided the real fabric for this book: Scilla Andreen-Hernandez, Audrey Bansmer, Robert Blackman, Karen Braverman, Bambi Breakstone, Molly Campbell, Brenda Cooper, Judith Curtis, Audrey Darin, Emily Draper, Lori Eskowitz, Nicole Gorsuch, Jenni Gullett, Bill Hargate, LuEllyn Harper, Kathleen Hillseth, Valerie Laven-Cooper, Darryl Levine, Brad Loman, Mona May, Debra McGuire, Louise Mingenbach, Elizabeth Palmer, Lynn Paolo, Erin Quigley, Melina Root, Charmaine Simmons, Marti Squires, Howard Sussman, Robert Turturice, Tony Velasco, and Jennifer von Mayrhaufer. They make it look so easy.

Introduction

What's on TV?

So many things, really: cops and robbers, doctors and lawyers, ancient gods and space aliens, nannies and professors, political candidates and journalists, young people in soft-focus love, old people in softer-focus love, scary people who do very bad stuff when you hear the creepy music start. Inside that magic box are dozens of disparate worlds, each spinning in its own special orbit. Now, despite the fact that you may believe a lawyer is totally different from a robber . . . umm, make that a doctor is totally different from an ancient god . . . okay, would you settle for a political candidate and an old person? Anyway. Despite the myriad cast of characters, there is a secret common denominator that unites them all in a single sphere, linking them together, making one indistinguishable from the next. And that mighty link answers to one name and one name only: Calvin Klein.

Or Donna Karan, or Hugo Boss, or GAP. On some shows, you can even see the softer side of Sears. Barring a few select cable-access channels, no matter where you look, you'll bear witness to a strange television phenomenon: *Everyone is wearing clothes*. Weird.

It's, like, a conspiracy or something. THE GOVERNMENT IS CENSORING OUR INALIENABLE RIGHT TO TOTAL NUDITY. Write your congressman! March! Strip!

Or just keep reading. Which is where we come into your face. Many experts assert that television is a barometer of popular taste, a reference point for the masses, even a vast cultural desert. Of course, if it were a desert, then it'd be hot, and they'd all be dressed like Bedouins, so clearly that's a stupid theory. (Nothing against you Bedouin readers out there—caftans are timeless!) To our minds, prime-time TV is an oasis of fashion tips, style ideas, and trend settings. It's a twenty-one-inch catalog that arrives fresh every day (not to be confused with the J. Crew catalog, which arrives every *other* day), chock full of designers, outfits for all climates and occasions, and models of varying body types. It's a place where you can sort through the racks until you find a look you want to make your own—or perhaps just borrow until the end of the season.

Then again, maybe you'd rather not burn precious viewing hours sorting through the racks. Maybe when you watch your favorite show you'd rather pay attention to, oh, say, the plot, or the jokes, or the creepy music so you know when to cover your eyes. True, clothes can sometimes be an integral part of the plotline. Think *Seinfeld.* Think *Cybill.* Think *The Nanny* (meanwhile, if you're doing so much thinking, why the hell are you watching *The Nanny*?). Generally, though, fashion statements don't surface in the script; rather, they subtly define a character's identity, occupation, and persona du jour. So subtly, in fact, that you might not notice that Helen Hunt never wears heels, or how John Lithgow always wears suspenders with a belt.

Which is where we come into your face—again. For nine solid months, we camped in front of our trusty Trinitrons, and fearlessly flipped from Gotham City to Lanford, Illinois, to Chicago, uh, Hope. At the end of the season, Val, who usually focuses on program substance over style, proudly announced that she'd noticed "lots of pretty Y-shaped necklaces and shiny vinyl stuff." Ellen, who favors network garb over gab, was astonished to discover that some shows are actually enjoyable *with the sound on.* These revelations in hand, we recruited the help of countless costume designers, stylists, hairdressers, and cable repairmen to compile the ultimate prime-time shopping guide: what to buy, where to buy it, how to make it—or even fake it.

To wit, in our never-ending quest to make your sartorial decisions easier, we've charted the small-screen fashion patterns so you wouldn't have to. So you could concentrate on the big picture and take in the details at your leisure. So you could go to the bathroom during commercials instead of sitting there like a couple of lamebrained writers, your legs clenched fiercely together, frantically scribbling notes, praying you didn't do any real damage to the couch before the news came on at eleven. No, no, don't give it a second thought. We love IKEA. It makes us feel like we're on the set of *Friends.*

What's on TV? Stay tuned.

Prime-Time Style

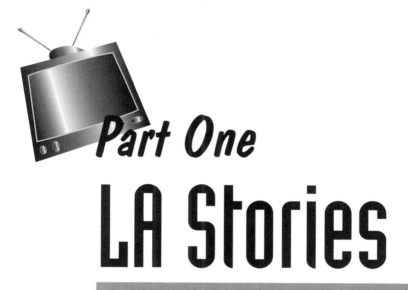

Part One

LA Stories

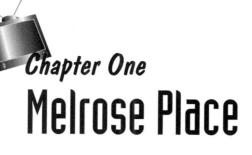

Chapter One
Melrose Place

MONDAY, 8:00 P.M. (FOX) MELROSE PLACE

(1992–present). Gritty, realistic drama about a dozen passingly attractive singles who live, work, and sleep together. Riveting hemlines, pastel plots, nuclear power suits. More blonding than bonding, but characters are dressed to kill—or at least disfigure. Go figure.

Welcome to Melrose Place, where the clothes are incredibly nice, and the people are . . . not. But who can blame them? They've been cast in crisis-driven drama—and on this show, there's no rest for the wicked. If your husband's not cheating on you, he's framing you for murder. If your wife's not blackmailing you, she's rising from the dead to possess your soul (don't you hate when that happens?). These people cannot catch a break. With all the sabotage and double-crossing, naturally they're psychopaths. With all the backstabbing and bloodshed, naturally they change outfits five times an episode. And with all the plate smashing and storming out of restaurants, naturally they're really, really thin. It only makes sense.

In fact it's the only thing that makes sense. Then again, what's a little suspension of disbelief between fabulously groomed friends? The unique beauty of *Melrose* is that you can always count on the characters to dress appropriately for every occasion: With every new mini-trauma, a new miniskirt; for every hangman, a lariat necklace. Whether they're attending a wedding, an office party, or a frontal lobotomy, Amanda & Co. can unfailingly throw together the perfect little outfit. Unlike us mere mortals, Melrosians never seem to angst over the true meaning of "black tie optional," or exactly how casual "casual Fridays" are meant to be, or how you're supposed to pull off a completely coordinated ensemble when you're faking blindness. It's, like, a gift.

Luckily, most gifts are made to be unwrapped (unless they're ticking, in which case RUN, SYDNEY, RUN LIKE THE WIND!). Below, some basic Melrose guidelines on dressing apropos of anything. Remember: If you can't beat 'em, fluff up your hair—and beat 'em harder.

So You Want to Commit a Murder....

Character to watch: Jane (Josie Bissett).

The situation: After being raped by Richard, Jane plots her revenge.

The look: Basic black.

Think: Audrey Hepburn in *Breakfast at Brentwood*.

The outfit: A black ribbed turtleneck, formfitting pants, and nylon mini–trench coat, topped off with a black knit cap. Hey, who's that? Oh, it's Jane in a black knit cap.

What else it could work for: Wandering around Soho. Shoplifting at the Louvre.

Most important accessory: Pretty silver gun—bullets optional.

In the larger scheme of things: Even when she's not packing heat, says Kathleen Hillseth, *Melrose*'s costumer, Jane favors formfitting pants—particularly the double-knit, hip-hugging Prada variety in brown, navy, and black (although they all look black on TV). Square-toed, square-heeled pull-on ankle boots are the footwear of choice. While not a big fan of dresses or skirts, when she does drop trou, she prefers short, A-line-ish skirts that hang low on her hips, with matching cropped jackets.

Finishing touches: A sheer chiffon kerchief around the neck knotted on the side (très Parisian), small diamond or pearl stud earrings (très subtle), and delicate lariat necklaces that look vintage (even if they're très nouveau).

The overall concept: "Since Jane's a clothing designer," says Hillseth, "we emphasize her fashion consciousness and make her the most cutting-edge of all the characters." On the color wheel, Hillseth keeps Josie Bissett out of reds and yellows to avoid making her already fair complexion look corpselike—the idea here is to look like the killer, not the killee.

Can you get away with it? The clothes or the crime? If, like Josie Bissett, you're short-waisted, long-limbed, and narrow-hipped, then yes—these are the clothes for you. And if, like Jane, you live in Melrose Place, again yes—in these parts, murder's a cinch.

So You Want to Be a Reluctant Accomplice to a Murder....

Character to watch: Sydney (Laura Leighton).

The situation: After Jane is raped by Richard, she discovers Sydney was the person who slipped her the mickey that temporarily paralyzed her last season. Armed with this knowledge, Jane blackmails Sydney to help her plot her revenge.

The look: Demented debutante in basic black.

Think: Cornelia Guest meets Pippi Longstocking. For lunch in Brentwood.

The outfit: See Jane. (See Jane run from Richard. See Sydney hit Richard on the head with a blunt object. See Richard fall down go boom.)

What else it could work for: Reluctantly helping someone wander around Soho. Reluctantly helping someone shoplift at the Louvre.

Most important accessory: Red hair peeking out from under black knit cap so viewers can tell you apart from the girl who's next to you wearing the exact same outfit.

In the larger scheme of things: Sydney changes her fashion philosophy almost as often as her alliances. In the past year, she's gone from Heidi Fleiss to Mary Quant to Mary Richards to Jackie O—making her closet a regular cornucopia of sleeveless dresses, Vivienne Tam ensembles, print pants, faux-Chanel suits, and go-go boots.

Finishing touches: Where to start? This dishy bird has more handbags than a bellboy—faux Prada, faux Hermès, faux Gucci (faux carrying her wallet, mascara, blackmail letters, and poison pills, of course). Plus, shoes, belts, headbands, bows, and poison pillbox hats to match.

The overall concept: Redheads have more fun. "We have a great time with Sydney," says Hillseth, "because we can experiment in so many different directions. She's the most over-the-top dresser, so we get to use really vivid colors on her—lots of lime greens and oranges and fuchsias—as well as crazy prints."

Can you get away with it? Do you have the ganglion stamina? More importantly, do you have a desk job?

So You Want to Stage a Corporate Coup and Then Go Bankrupt . . .

Character to watch: Richard (Patrick Muldoon).

The situation: After Richard is rejected by Jane, he plots his revenge and ousts her from their joint business venture. Jane, in turn, plots her revenge and sabotages his fashion show by setting off the fire sprinklers. Richard goes bankrupt and plots his revenge—anew!

The look: Tall, dark, whistle-slick, and dressed to the gills—except during bankruptcy, when he lapsed into plaid flannel for five whole minutes.

Think: Dracula meets Armani—with a brief howdy-do to Lamar Alexander.

The outfit: A three-button suit, so finely tailored it sets your teeth on edge.

What else it could work for: George Hamilton's funeral.

Most important accessory: The metaphorical pistol in his pocket (although he'll *claim* he's just glad to see you).

In the larger scheme of things: Richard means business and dresses accordingly. No casual Joe, even his pajamas probably have pinstripes. He's dark, pressed, and starched—and so are his clothes.

Finishing touches: The occasional collarless shirt, French cuffs, a terminal smirk.

The overall concept: According to Tony Velasco, costumer for the *Melrose* men, "We want Richard to epitomize what young men are wearing in the business world." Translation: We want Richard to epitomize what we hazily imagine young men are wearing in the business world. In other words, Richard struts around in Calvin Klein and Hugo Boss while those poor schlubs in the bullpen known as Real Life sweat through their Brooks Brothers potato sacks.

Can you get away with it? Sure, although the terminal smirk part could get you slapped on the subway.

So You Want to Have an Amphetamine Addiction . . .

Character to watch: Matt (Doug Savant).

The situation: After too many all-night studying sessions, gay medical student Matt turns to artificial stimulants for help—and his nervous system plots its revenge.

The look: Land's meets End.

Think: So not pink.

The outfit: A mess of clothing from GAP that's been slept in for three days.

What else it could work for: Law school.

Most important accessory: A key to the hospital pharmacy.

In the larger scheme of things: What larger scheme of things? Pile together a big bunch of khakis, sweatshirts, distressed jeans, sneakers, and T-shirts, and you're full speed ahead.

Finishing touches: Rumpled hair, a slightly wild-eyed look.

The overall concept: ZZZZZzzz.

Can you get away with it? Yeah, but it's a look that burns out fast.

So You Want to Get Married Behind Bars . . .

Prison bars, that is.

Character to watch: Amanda (Heather Locklear).

The situation: After Peter is wrongly accused of murder, Amanda hastily arranges a jailhouse wedding so she won't have to testify at his trial, only to find out that the actual Dr. Peter Burns may not be the man she married. Forthwith, she—and say it with us, won't you—*plots her revenge.*

The look: Nuptial blitz.

Think: Debbie Does Matrimony.

The outfit: A too, too short, off-off white fitted dress with matching sandals.

What else it could work for: Debbie Does Registered Nursing.

Most important accessory: The weepy prison guards in the background.

In the larger scheme of things: With her propensity for short and tight, Amanda—via Gucci, Versace, and Bebe—drastically redefined the power suit. Since Heather Locklear isn't crazy about her knees, she leans toward sky-high hemlines (we didn't really follow the logic, either, but whatever). Her matching jackets are nipped, cinched, and buttoned within a millimeter of their lives. As for shoes, Locklear would rather go without entirely. "She sticks with shoes that are easy to put on and take off, like Donna Karan heels, sandals, or mules," says Hillseth. "She'll only wear them in scenes where you can see her feet. Otherwise, she walks around in her own slippers." Out of the office, Amanda dons Levi's 501s, baby Ts, ballet sweaters, and scoop-neck tanks. And on formal occasions, she takes the light, tight, sleeveless, backless route.

Finishing touches: Pale lips, frothy lingerie, Pamela Barish gold-and-purple velvet bathrobe, men's pajamas, stud earrings.

The overall concept: Tough and teeny. Locklear fits a size two—but only if it's been taken in. "She's so small," says Hillseth, "it's hard to find pants that fit her. Also, she has no butt—if she drops as little as three pounds, it makes a difference. We have to alter everything so she doesn't look too skinny." The poor dear. Palette-wise, Amanda walks a lighter shade of pale: lilac, celery,

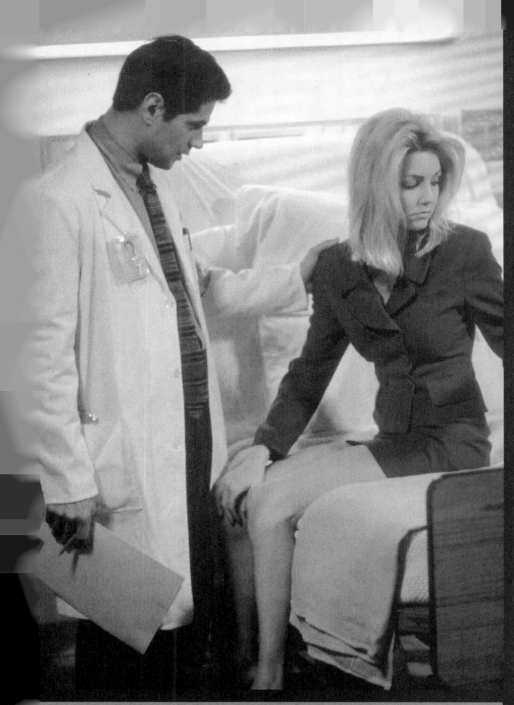

Even power suits need tune-ups now and then. With a skirt that tight, it's no wonder Amanda (Heather Locklear, sitting right) needed to pay a visit to Dr. Michael Mancini (Thomas Calabro). Is there a hair-colorist in the house?

sky blue, baby pink, buttercup—no grays or tans allowed. "We use red for a statement color," says Hillseth. "She wears it in scenes where she needs to come across especially strong."

Can you get away with it? If you're extremely wee, *mais oui*.

So You Want to Be a Multiple Personality . . .

Character to watch: Kimberly (Marcia Cross).

The situation: After remarrying Michael, Kimberly is happy at last—and in light of this unacceptable condition, alter egos Rita and Betsy make it their business to plot Kimberly's revenge.

The look: Changes all the time.

Think: Fast!

The outfit: A short-sleeved ribbed turtleneck atop a long straight skirt . . . make that black jeans and a tank with a black motorcycle jacket . . . no, a Laura Ashley floral print dress with matching headband and flat shoes . . . she can't decide. And neither can she. *And neither can she.*

What else it could work for: The typical urban professional/biker chick/Junior Leaguer. You know, the girls next door.

Most important accessory: Multiple shoe trees.

In the larger scheme of things: When Kimberly's feeling like herself, she wears generic cropped sweaters and jeans, straight skirts both long and short, and tailored trousers. When she's feeling a little depressed, she'll fall back on unstructured blouses, roomy, comfy sweaters, and jeans or leggings. When she's feeling a little Rita, she does the heavy metal mamba. And when she's feeling a little Betsy, she's the Tupperware Princess of Chintz.

Finishing touches: A long, gold satin Donna Karan peignoir set, Only Hearts red bra and panties, and other assorted naughty niceties (for Kimberly). Matronly handbags, perky headbands, and innocent flannel nightgowns (for Betsy). An invisible Harley-Davidson (for Rita).

The overall concept: You are what you wear. "Marcia Cross likes playing multiple personalities," says Hillseth, "because it puts her in specific costumes. She doesn't have to think about her clothes, and this frees her to concentrate on her acting." Wait a minute. What do you mean, *acting*???

Can you get away with it? Mmm . . . hard to say. The odds are three to one.

So You Want to Be Committed to a Mental Institution . . .

Character to watch: Peter (Jack Wagner).

The situation: After being wrongfully accused of murder, Peter takes his only alibi, Kimberly, to the police station to vouch for his innocence. En route, Kimberly morphs into Betsy, drugs him, commits him to a mental institution, and prescribes several rounds of intense electro-shock therapy with a lobotomy chaser. Battered but not quite beaten, Peter feebly struggles to remember what it was that he meant to plot.

The look: I've fallen and I can't get up.

Think: Ken Doll meets Ken Kesey.

The outfit: Hospital gown with a peek-a-boo back and matching slippers.

What else it could work for: Oh, say, a flashback on *General Hospital.*

Most important accessory: Extra-long sleeves that tie around the back.

In the larger scheme of things: When in his more usual uncommitted state, Peter makes a much smarter impression. "He's almost always in a suit," says Velasco. "We like to keep his look sharp—pin-striped suits with double-breasted jackets in lighter tones, and white shirts." On the weekends, he's a Ralph Lauren slacks and polo-shirt man.

Finishing touches: A short burgundy silk bathrobe for those special moments when Dr. Burns turns up the heat.

The overall concept: A lean, preen fighting machine.

Can you get away with it? It's your diagnosis—the clothes are easy, but the attitude's a tricky dick.

So You Want to Spring Someone from a Mental Institution . . .

Character to watch: Michael (Thomas Calabro).

The situation: After learning of Kimberly and Peter's disappearance, Michael and Amanda set off to search for them. Tips lead them to the mental institution, where they break through a locked window, elude shrieking inmates and orderlies, and save Peter just seconds under the lobotomy wire. In the ensuing tussle, Kimberly nearly dies, and this sobering experience causes Michael to reassess his insidious revenge-plotting ways.

The look: Satan takes a holiday.

Think: Dr. Demento turns over a new leaf.

The outfit: Jeans and a navy blue V-necked sweater.

What else it could work for: Club MeD.

Most important accessory: Tuft of manly chest hair.

In the larger scheme of things: For years, Michael has been *Melrose*'s resident villain. "We put him in dark, monochromatic sport coats, slacks, and ties," says Velasco. "He's not as formal as Peter, but he still maintains a professional appearance with unbuttoned single-breasted jackets over darker-hued shirts—never white."

Finishing touches: Due to Michael's highly personal bedside manner, he's frequently caught with his pants down. Hence, bulk shipments of Calvin Klein boxers.

The overall concept: Is there a viper in the house? And where did he get those snappy clothes?

Can you get away with it? Yessssssssss.

So You Want to Be Possessed by the Spirit of Your Dead Wife . . .

Character to watch: Billy (Andrew Shue).

The situation: After Brooke's attempted suicide, Billy continues to push her for a divorce, which pushes her right over the edge. Of the pool. She drowns and her spirit miraculously rises from the mosaic tiles to set up temporary residence in Billy's body. Billy becomes the woman he married and proceeds to plot his spirit guide's metaphysical revenge.

The look: Your worst preppie nightmare.

Think: Andrew Shue demands that his contract specify expansion of boring-ass character.

The outfit: Chinos, a casual shirt, and an expression of sheer terror.

What else it could work for: A German tourist in Miami.

Most important accessory: A cross and several cloves of garlic.

In the larger scheme of things: Pre-soul-possession, fair-minded Billy was a Dockers kind of guy—white button-down shirts, bright ties, polo shirts, plaid prints, jeans, and sneakers or loafers. Post-soul-possession, back-stabbing Billy edged toward the dark side. When evil proved to be the root of all money, he found he could afford more stylish clothes in more ominous colors—suits and European-tailored sport coats in black, brown, and charcoal, and Australian gator boots. Funny how that works.

Finishing touches: A startling lack of acting ability—but, hey, he went to Dartmouth.

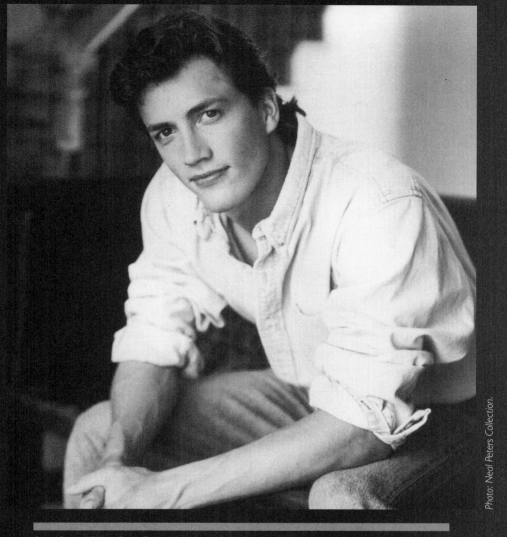

See Good Billy. See Good Billy sit. See Good Billy smile. He is not Bad Billy. Good Billy wears a white shirt and jeans. Bad Billy does not. Bad Billy is very, very bad. Smile, Good Billy, smile!

The overall concept: Andrew Shue demands that his contract specify expansion of boring-ass wardrobe.

Can you get away with it? Depends. How good is your agent?

So You Want to Be Widowed at an Incredibly Young Age . . .

Character to watch: Alison (Courtney Thorne-Smith).

The situation: After much-beleaguered recovering alcoholic Alison marries ex-millionaire Hayley, his debts force them to flee the country on his last remaining yacht. Late one night, she gets out of bed to look for her new husband, only to discover that he's hit rock bottom. Literally. Sad and lonely, she falls off the wagon, quits her job, and takes a break from the rat race to try to sort out this whole revenge-plotting thing.

The look: A pajama party on the *Titanic.*

Think: The captain and chenille.

The outfit: That famous Damze chenille bathrobe (moon-and-stars pattern), which has covered more bare skin than John Tesh's hair plugs.

What else it could work for: What else *couldn't* it work for? It's already been on *The Nanny, Frasier, Baywatch, NYPD Blue, Lois and Clark, Friends, Murphy Brown,* and *Beverly Hills, 90210.* This is the bathrobe that never sleeps.

Most important accessory: Toll-free order number for Damze.

In the larger scheme of things: Alison is the girl most likely to wear clothes that regular people might actually wear, too. By day, she sports streamlined separates (à la Calvin Klein or Agnes B.)— pin-striped straight skirts, turtlenecks, jewel-necked tops, and sleeveless dresses with jackets. By night, she kicks around in leggings and sweatshirts, jeans, and baby Ts. No painfully strappy sandals for this girl; heeled loafers or sneakers suit her fine.

Finishing touches: Small jewelry, lariat necklaces, cozy wool socks and comfy undershirts for lounging at home.

The overall concept: Classic, simple, normal, relaxed, earnest, and really so very well meaning.

Can you get away with it? Of course you can! You can do anything you set your mind to!

So You Want to Save the Day . . .

Character to watch: Jake (Grant Show).

The situation: After Alison, Sydney, and Matt find themselves jobless, good ol' reliable Jake is ready to bail them out with a job at his bar, Shooters, so they can make the rent and plot their revenues (gotcha!).

The look: Rugged, yet tidy.

Think: The Marlboro Man quits smoking.

The outfit: Levi's Silver Tab jeans, white T-shirt under a plaid shirt. All-cotton, buttoned up, and tucked in, natch.

What else it could work for: Escape to Walton's Mountain.

Most important accessory: An employees' Shooters T-shirt and apron extended in one hand, while other hand pats unhappy-character-of-the-month on the back.

In the larger scheme of things: Denim, plaid, motorcycle boots, Timberland boots, tennis shoes, Nikes, chambray work shirts, duck-hunting jackets. Jake owns one suit: a single-breasted gabardine Donna Karan number under which he wears—guess what—a T-shirt.

Finishing touches: A leather motorcycle jacket to tell you he has a dangerous side, a good watch to tell you he has the time.

The overall concept: Nice guys never wear ties.

Can you get away with it? With what—being the only good apple in a rotten bushel? Please. If you want to save the day, you're in

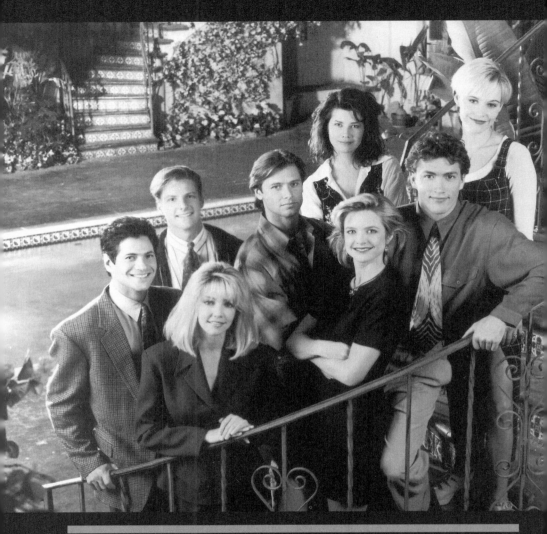

Say cheese. The Original Melrose Eight poses by the cleanest pool in America (ever notice how there's always a maintenance man skimming the surface? All those condoms probably clog the drainage system). Clockwise from the blonde with the shortest hair: Pretty perky Jane (Josie Bissett) whistles pixie in neo-Liederhosen jumper; Big bad Billy (Andrew Shue) draws psychotic patterns—even around his neck; Pooh-pooh Alison (Courtney Thorne-Smith) makes a classic, conservative stand; HRH Amanda (Heather Locklear) suits herself to power; Not-so-nasty Michael (Thomas Calabro) checks in with casual yet professional style; Door-Matt (Doug Savant) shows his stripes in a tie *and a windbreaker*; St. Jake (Grant Show) is forever plaid; and Jo (Daphne Zuniga) is, at this point, a mere figment of Jake's imagination. Not seen at bottom of pool: Brooke.

the wrong place. Better to pack your squeaky-clean bags and march on over to ***Beverly Hills, 90210***. Which, coincidentally, is just where we're headed. Don't forget to look both ways before you turn the page.

Melrose Dos—and Don'ts

Looking for a little trim? Then you're in the right place. If there's one thing all the overworked *Melrose* hairstyles have in common, it's that they require constant upkeep, supervision, and bleach. Like the pool. We consulted three tress-experts—Steven Berg, a stylist at Manhattan's John Barrett Salon, Kim Lepine, owner of Kim Lepine Hair Salon, and Grant McCracken, Ph.D., an anthropologist and author of *Big Hair*—to analyze how Melrosians make the cut. Below, the characters with the most buck for their bangs. Comb on.

Amanda (Heather Locklear): The unanimous verdict: Busy as a little beaver. "It's too moppish; it should be cleaned up," said Lepine. "She has a little bit of everyone on her head," said Berg, "Jennifer Aniston's crown, Courteney Cox's bangs, Goldie Hawn's layers—with a dash of Morgan Fairchild thrown in." In keeping with her personality, however, the chaos is tightly controlled. "It may *look* like just-out-of-bed hair," said McCracken, "but it takes work to get that level of polish. The fact that it's so high-maintenance reflects Amanda's meticulously managed life." What would our experts call this style? "Over," said Berg.

Jane (Josie Bissett): Praise ran high for Jane's pixie cut. "It's perfect," enthused Berg. "The dark roots work—she'd look too processed without them. She's got stringy hair, which is limiting;

you can't do much else with it. But it's a cut that takes nerve; not every girl could carry it off." The only drawback, McCracken pointed out, is that "it doesn't give her an air of authority. It's winning and fashionable, but it won't help her get taken seriously." Then again, he added, "it's a good cover for her hostile intent to hurt Richard." What kind of statement does this style make? Quoth Berg: "I want to be in Wilson Phillips."

Peter (Jack Wagner): With a little color-lightening, Lepine thought this coif would be just right. "It's natural," she said. "The layers work well with his face." Berg liked that the style has no definite part, which makes it more updated. "It's Jake's haircut, six months later," he said. The overall effect: "Perfectly unperfect."

Sydney (Laura Leighton): Regarding Sydney, "She's chopped and layered all over the place," said McCracken. "Just like her character." Commented Lepine, "It's cute in a retro-sixties way, but she should modernize it by throwing in streaks—the single-process dying is flat." Berg felt it was trendy, but a tad too done. "She's got the bubble happening up top, the poofy crown, the flippy bottom, and the whole back is layered. It's Teri Hatcher's hair, grown out."

Jake (Grant Show): Lepine calls this the gladiator cut; Berg labeled it a combed-down Caesar. (We think they're splitting hairs.) "It's masculine without being doltish," said McCracken. Berg, on the other hand, deemed Jake "a fashion victim—everyone else on TV had short hair, so he got his shorn, too." The upshot? "It's the look of a guy whose girlfriend dragged him to her hairdresser," observed Berg. "It's an 'against my will' haircut."

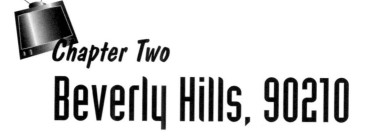

Chapter Two
Beverly Hills, 90210

WEDNESDAY, 8:00 P.M. (FOX) BEVERLY HILLS, 90210

(1990–present). Classic college coming-of-age romp with heartwarming school-day fare: romances lost and found, varsity rivalries, battering boyfriends, homicidal roommates, junkie love, and the like. Earnest presentation of major fashion issues, nondiscriminatory use of vinyl, dyed-to-match mini-backpacks and banners. Ever so touching.

Whereas the residents of *Melrose Place* are suited for revenge, the students at *90210*'s California University prefer to wear their ethics on their sleeves. This is serious dressing with a cause on the side—a homecoming parade of current moral *cum* sartorial trends. Brandon and the gang are PC beyond belief. Oooh, goody, pop quiz:

> On *90210*, the abbreviation PC stands for:
> (a) Politically Correct
> (b) Prettily Clothed
> (c) Peculiarly Coifed
> (d) All of the above

D, All of the above. These righteous do-gooders leave no stone unturned, no injustice unfought, no belly button unbared. They don't shoot up at the Viper Room, they link pinkies at the Peach Pit. They don't gossip, they intervene. They can't just go to the bathroom, they have *movements*. They don't air-kiss, they group-hug and say, "I love you guys!" Frankly, if they didn't have such cool accessories and great cars, they'd make us spew chunks. Which is yet another example of how skillful costuming can transform a bunch of namby-pamby L7s into really well dressed people with passion and integrity. Yup. It's like magic.

In the meantime, you can embrace their cause with their clothing . . . or ditch the cause and just take the clothing . . . or keep the cause and go naked to protest the exploitation of twelve-year-old Honduran sweatshop workers sewing their little fingers to the bone for thirty cents a day because craven, overfed Americans want more, more, more for less, less . . . anyway. As usual, it's completely your right to choose. Would that this were always the case.

Take Back the Brights

Our agenda: To liberate the public from the oppressive bummer grip of all-black clothing and raise the color consciousness of the masses to peak neon levels. This is not the time to be neutral! Just say no to drabs! *Hue* can make a difference!

Committee members: Claire, Donna, Steve.

Progress report: To date, Claire (Kathleen Robertson) has effectively utilized her art history major to mix color where no color has mixed before. She's currently focusing on our "Code Red" project, venturing forth in hot pinks, bright reds, and vivid violets. According to committee chairperson (*90210* costume designer) Molly Campbell, Claire's dark hair and pale skin make her an ideal candidate for saturated tones. In addition, Claire has begun to experiment with prints. Since patterns often don't translate well on television, however, we are not convinced this is the most strategic method of delivering our message. A vote will be held at the end of the meeting to determine our future policy regarding this issue.

On the Jelly Bean platform, Donna (Tori Spelling) reports great success. Thus far, lime greens, raspberry reds, lemon yellows, and bubble gum pinks have cooperated nicely with her champagne hair and tan complexion. Our polls indicate that her symbolic blend of neutrals and brights—for example, brown showing through chartreuse, or gray under fuchsia—powerfully expresses our favorite party line: "Don't be dull—bedazzle!"

In a more subtle campaign, Steve (Ian Ziering) is raising the color consciousness of his fraternity set with intensified pastels. His impassioned use of lavender, royal blue, and mint green demonstrates that inside every male student body is a rainbow crying to get out. We have high hopes that Steve will come through with his promise to free ROY G BIV by the end of the year.

Final notes: Donna's proposal that we adjourn each meeting with a committee group hug and "I Love You Guys" cheer was met with unanimous agreement. We'll start this up next week. See you there!

Protect Our Right to Bare Arms

Our motto: A well-ventilated aesthetic, being necessary to the comfort of a high-temperature state, the right of the people to bare arms—and legs and chests and midriffs—shall not be infringed.

Committee members: Donna, Claire, Kelly, Steve.

Progress report: Committee consensus appears to be splintering, due to a difference in opinion on how best to achieve our goals. On the left, Donna asserts that the quickest way to make inroads is through maximum exposure. To this end, she supports skinny minis, unprotected navels, halter tops, and sleeveless shifts. In her defense, Molly Campbell declares, "She's got incredibly long, slim legs, a gorgeous tan, and she's a courageous dresser. Naturally she's going to show skin." Or should we say au naturelly? At any rate, plunging necklines and platform sandals confirm that Donna can divest her torso—and more so.

On the right, Kelly (Jennie Garth) prefers to wear cropped T-shirts, which cast a shadow over her stomach, thus creating the *illusion* of bareness. She is judicial, too, with her gam disclosure, choosing mid-thigh over mid-crotch hemlines. She'd rather go sleeveless than legless or belly-less (and wouldn't we all?); her style bespeaks her conviction that we must assimilate slowly to avoid any shocks to the system.

Mid-rift, Claire and Steve function as liaisons between camps. Claire mediates in the occasional belly-baring ensemble or micro-mini with navy baby Ts, and foot-flaunting strappy, high-heeled sandals. Steve flexes his crusading muscle in vests by Remy. Even with a T-shirt underneath, his vests are a great way for men all over campus to show a little skin without uncovering too much unsightly body hair. He's also dabbling in formal-wear via a spread-collar dress shirt by Emporio Armani (hey, that's a whole extra half-inch of neck skin flapping out there!). Steve and Claire are assiduously making efforts to unite our party platform with as little friction as possible. Because, seriously—who needs ugly chafing?

Final notes: Our ski weekend in Tahoe was canceled due to extreme cold and terrible skin-baring conditions. Fortunately, the I Love You Guys SPF 25 is finally available. See you Nair!

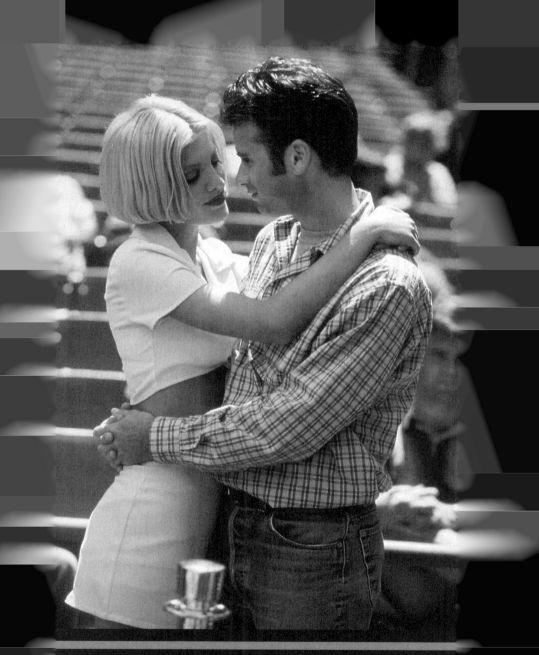

Oh, Ray. Little Ray. Remember when you used to be my boyfriend? And the way you used to hit me? Do you like my outfit, Ray? Isn't it amazing how all the money in Beverly Hills can't buy a girl good taste in clothing? Or a good dye-job, for that matter? Still, I have a pretty stomach, don't I, Ray? Uh-huh. You can look, but you can't touch. That's right, Ray. Some things

Recycle for a Better Tomorrow

Our agenda: To put an end to the shameful waste of valuable fashion styles from the past and revive the looks of our fore-siblings so they may be preserved for posterity. In with the old! Out with the new! Find your place in history—today!

Committee members: Brandon, Kelly.

Progress report: We're sad to see that President Brandon's (Jason Priestley) term has come to an end. Since that whole fiasco when he became student body president, he's had it with politics and plans to concentrate on his journalistic endeavors. Besides which, he claims passing the torch is prudent at this juncture in the movement. Whatever. We salute his incredible impact on the fight to wear period pieces, in the form of 1940s hand-painted silk ties, 1950s-style J. Crew chinos, and stiff Big Star ink jeans. We'd also like to note that despite the *sturm und drang* (German 101) around him, he's never strayed far from neutral earth tones and dark-hued basic button-down shirts. What *und* rock. Evoking the spirit of James Dean, Brandon is our very own rebel with a cause.

Taking over as our leader is Kelly. Just out of rehab and centered beyond belief, she vows to continue in the 1950s vein. As a womyn, Kelly will present fresh perspectives on this look with pale, highly feminine suits, as well as pastel mohair sweater sets and pearls. Campbell reminds us of Kelly's commitment to dresses over trousers, preferably simple silk sheaths, flowing rayon skirts, or straight-to-the-ankle columns of crepe. When she does venture into trouser territory, she opts for Armani stretch pants. With the utmost grace, Kelly promises to raise retro consciousness to a noon high.

Final notes: Our special farewell party for Brandon will be held at the Peach Pit. A sign-up sheet for the I Love You Guys karaoke committee is now posted on the bulletin board. Do, re, mi, fa, so, la, see you there!

Be a *90210*-ster—or just look like one.

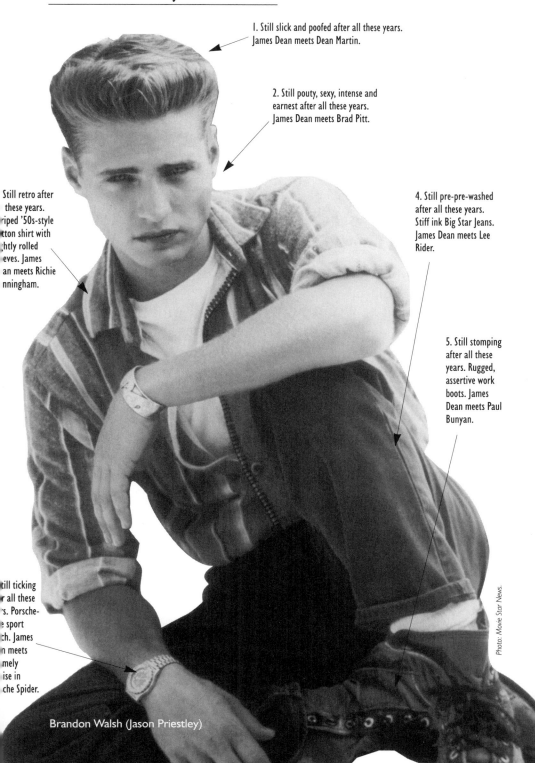

1. Still slick and poofed after all these years. James Dean meets Dean Martin.

2. Still pouty, sexy, intense and earnest after all these years. James Dean meets Brad Pitt.

Still retro after these years. riped '50s-style tton shirt with htly rolled eves. James an meets Richie nningham.

4. Still pre-pre-washed after all these years. Stiff ink Big Star Jeans. James Dean meets Lee Rider.

5. Still stomping after all these years. Rugged, assertive work boots. James Dean meets Paul Bunyan.

till ticking r all these rs. Porsche- e sport ch. James n meets mely ise in che Spider.

Brandon Walsh (Jason Priestley)

Photo: Movie Star News.

One Giant Step for Personkind

Our agenda: To walk the earth with sure foot and square heel, leaving our imprints on society without treading upon the rights and values of those who stride among us. Right! Left! Right, left, right!

Committee members: Brandon, David, Steve, Donna, Claire.

Progress report: A march is tentatively slated for November sweeps week (okay, so it'll be our 243rd march of the season, but how else are we supposed to drum up support? Hold a bake sale?). Once again, our promotional sponsors—Nike, Reebok, and Converse—will make their athletic footwear available to anyone interested.

We'll organize our march in the conventional manner: Brandon has agreed to get a toehold in Clarks and traditional English oxfords and wingtips. Steve will fall into step with cowboy boots and sneakers. Per usual, David (Brian Austin Green) will supply the music. He'll represent the trend set, complementing his monochromatic Tommy Hilfiger street style with chunky Adidas sneakers and Doc Martens.

Final notes: A vote was taken and our consensus was that enlisting female members is a must for next season. Also, the I Love You Guys (not *love* as in *love*, but *love* as in *like*) picket signs for the march have been assembled. See you, *frère!*

Save a Cotton Bush—Wear Synthetics

Our agenda: To prevent the mindless slaughter of innocent cotton plants, the barbaric shearing of really cold sheep, and the ruthless genocide of overworked silkworms. Don't waste a cotton-picking moment! Don't let them pull the wool over your eyes! Just because worms are slimy and gross doesn't mean they don't have itty-bitty feelings, too!

Committee members: Donna, Claire.

Progress report: Recruitment remains a problem. Donna is striving hard to cultivate grassroots support, but with minimum results. Still, no matter how many natural fiber–philes she encounters, she continues to log in the man(made)-hours. Most recently, Donna is retreading her "Rubber: It's Not Just for Tires Anymore" speech for the next campus rally. She intends to state her case in a red rubber sleeveless mini-dress, making her faux agenda *très vrai* indeed.

Claire is canvassing door-to-door in an attempt to increase membership. Early returns are disappointing: most dorm denizens still associate vinyl with their old LPs, and are reluctant to espouse the shiny black hip-huggers that espouse Claire. Nor has there been much enthusiasm for Claire's Spandex or Lycra body suits and leggings. At last report, a dozen-odd frat brothers roundly applauded Claire for her pink polyester jumpsuit, but when asked to join the fight to save our natural resources, they laughed, crushed beer cans against their foreheads, and belched negatory.

Final notes: A protest at the local GAP store is scheduled for next weekend. Acrylic scarves bearing the I Love You Guys logo will be distributed prior to our Sheep Liberation Day festivities. See ewe there!

Links Across America

Our agenda: To extend the chains of love, find a bead of truth, and join hands in a golden circle of peace and goodwill, thus making the world a shinier, more sparkly place to live in. Stick your neck out! Let freedom ring! Buy lots of jewelry!

Committee members: Claire, Donna, Kelly, David.

Progress report: Great news! Kelly managed to infiltrate the mainstream with her silver barbed-wire heart necklace designed by Hal Ludicer, and the message has reached all the way to MTV in NYC. On a bigger yet smaller note, Kelly is wearing delicate crystal lariat and add-a-bead necklaces. She also takes a shine to Hal Ludicer's stacked rings, and teensy-weensy earrings. According to Campbell, oversized earrings just don't cut it when you're trying to change the world, because "large, swinging earrings are distracting on close-ups." So true.

A mix of vintage pieces with contemporary jewelry from Sonia Ootin and Joan Goldman allows Claire to link the past with the future of our movement. She's also pushing the Hal Ludicer concept, with lots of silver necklaces and earrings. "Silver is bigger than gold right now," says Campbell, "but there's a trend back toward gold-chain combinations with gold charms." At wrist level, Claire's been spotted wearing a pair of very heavy chunky steel bangles that lock shut with a key and are connected by a sturdy chain. Talk about your Bond girls. And David's music-world connections keep him well ornamented in gold-chain necklaces, or leather necklaces with beads. Oh, he may sport a single gold-hoop earring, but he'll always be a stud to us.

Final notes: Our special I. (as in, I Love You Guys) D. (dearly) bracelets will be sold at the bookstore for a limited time. C. U. there!

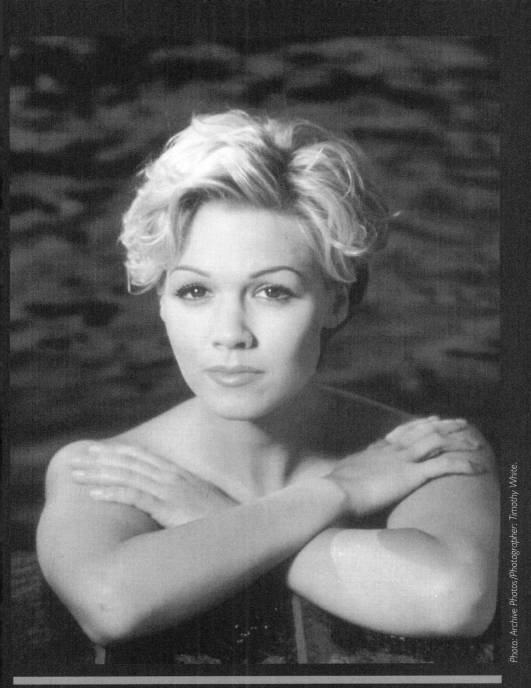

90210's Kelly (Jennie Garth) takes a breather—and for good reason. Every female character on the show has at least five costume changes per episode. No wonder her hair looks

Hell No—I Won't Go

Agenda: Count me way out.

Committee members: Valerie

Progress report: As anticipated, Valerie (Tiffani-Amber Thiessen) has firmly upheld her credo that she would join no club that would have "that stupid Kelly" as a member. Val's primary goal is to keep her life and style as far from "that perky do-gooder Donna" as possible. She furthers her separation from "that moronic gang" by accessorizing with a scowl and arched eyebrow; given a different zip code, she'd throw in the finger, too. Since she endeavors to be cooler, more dangerous, and more experienced (i.e., at all cool, at all dangerous, experienced in any way whatsoever), she distinguishes herself from "that loser Brady Bunch" by wearing edgier styles in darker colors. "She's a brunette with olive skin, so she looks wonderful in chocolate browns and neutral earth tones," says Campbell, her closest ally. "She has a sophisticated silhouette with tailored, fitted jackets, black cigarette pants, knits, and short-sleeved sweaters." To confuse her enemies, Valerie might don a sleeveless, deceivingly innocent white dress. But don't be fooled: the only thing that can sway her multifarious nefarious efforts is the distraction of some drug-sniffin', law-runnin' Dylan, Colin, or Harryin', whose predilection for dark tones meshes with her own.

Final notes: Plans for an "I Love Other People's Guys" tattoo are under way on Valerie's butt. See you . . . there?

Or better yet, let's blow this clothes-conscious network, make tracks for the City of Sin-dication, and watch some serious bay. Get it? Bay + Watch = *Baywatch*. See? ***Baywatch***. It's okay, Yasmine—don't fret your cute little self over this hard math stuff. You just go to the next chapter and look at the pretty pictures. Uh-huh. That's you! Pretty!

Fashion Statements You'll Never Hear on *90210*

"Loving that fur coat!"

"Honestly, Donna, put on a looser pair of pants—they're so tight, you can practically see the outline of your cervical cap."

"Meanwhile, I saw the cutest twin set on a woman at the welfare office!"

"I can't—I'm late to meet David at Chess King."

"Go with the fluorescent shirt—that way when you drive home stinking high, other drivers can see you better."

"Loving those leg warmers!"

"Do you think a nipple ring hurts?"

"Meanwhile, I saw the cutest shoes on some girl in the waiting room of the abortion clinic!"

"Oh, just wear any old thing."

"Yeah, it's a great swimsuit, but that girl so obviously has fake boobs. Frankly, I just can't get behind something like that."

"Loving that smoking jacket!"

"Meanwhile, I saw the cutest vintage coat on some guy at the needle exchange!"

"You don't like my skirt? *Fuck you!*"

"Don't you adore these earrings? I'm telling you, shoplifting's the way to go!"

"Nah—too short."

Chapter Three

Baywatch

SATURDAY, 7:00 P.M. (SYNDICATED) **BAYWATCH**

(1989–present). Surf 'n' turf adventures involving lissome crew of life-guards in waterproof mascara. Major maillot, bikini, and trunk show—they jump, jiggle, jog, and jet-ski, all for the common good. Sand gets in your eyes.

I f on *Melrose* they dress for the occasion, on *Baywatch*, they dress . . . occasionally. And if on *90210* they dress for a cause, on *Baywatch*, they dress, just . . . 'cause. 'Cause in most countries, total nudity is illegal on non-cable television channels. 'Cause if they didn't, there'd be no reason to scope out Pamela Lee's romantic honeymoon video. 'Cause scant bits of fabric stretched over bodacious female bodies is a universal language—hence, international popularity! So many reasons, really. Below, the top five *Baywatch* 'Cause and effects.

'Cause Everyone Suits Up Differently

On *Baywatch*, no two swimsuits are alike. Now, you might be thinking, "What in the Sam Hill are Val and Ellen talking about? Aren't those red lifeguard uniforms standard issue? Doesn't the Coast Guard regulate this stuff?" To which we reply: Hello! Like

Knightrider had anything to do with highway patrol? *This is television.* According to Karen Braverman, *Baywatch*'s costume designer, "Although the front of every lifeguard suit looks exactly the same, in actuality, they're very different. Each suit is custom-made and measured to each girl's body type." The moral: You can't judge a "book" by its cover.

And now you might be thinking, "What in the Sam Hill are Val and Ellen trying to put over on us? They all have the same body type: perfect. How many types of perfection can there be?" To which we reply: Hello! Like we're personally acquainted with physical perfection? *We're not the ones on television.* The only hypothesis we can draw here is that perfection apparently has a range of requirements. For instance, C. J. (Pamela Anderson Lee—PAL!) and Neely (Gena Lee Nolin) save lives in maillots with deep scoop fronts, deeper scoop backs, and French-cut legs—all the better to execute their courageous cleavage mission. Stephanie (Alexandra Paul) polices the beach in lingerie straps and high-cut legs—all the better to accomplish her daring sculptured-shoulder mission. Caroline (Yasmine Bleeth) stands sentinel in a scoop-front, crisscross back, and, again, French-cut legs—all the better to carry out her intrepid look-at-my-pretty-back mission. In addition, some of the actresses opt for fuller linings in their suit fronts to provide extra support. And while Braverman refused to name names, she did verify that PAL was not one of those women.

Off duty, the perfection range becomes even more varied. C. J. fritters away her frolic hours in triangle-top, Brazilian-cut bottomed bikinis. "Her suits are formfitting and small; they don't use a lot of material," says Braverman. "Pamela usually wears white; it shows off her wonderful tan. She's a minimalist." Make that micromalist. Along the same minuscule lines, Caroline sand-cruises in Brazilian-cut bikini bottoms, although the matching halter-cut tops are often equipped with underwire control. In contrast, Stephanie leans toward one-piecers with high necks, racer backs, and cutaway arms

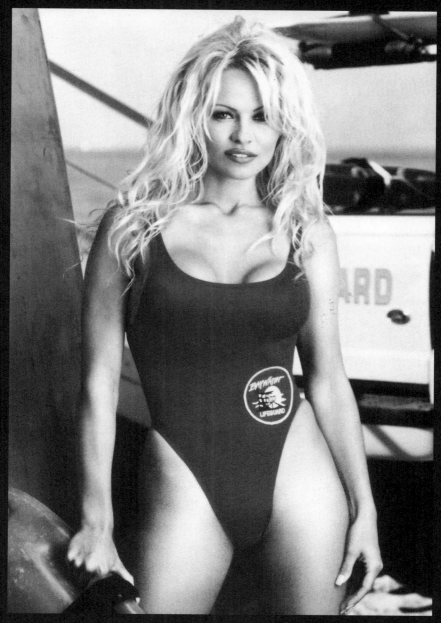

Baywatch's Pamela Anderson Lee in her standard issue (yeah, right) regulation maillot. She romps, she rescues, she resuscitates.

"to accentuate her tall, lean, athletic body," explains Braverman. And last but not least (well, maybe next to least), Neely freely wheelies in teeny, weeny revealy bikinis. Say *that* ten times fast.

Which brings us to the *Baywatch* men (they would be the ones with body hair and no boobs). On the job, Mitch (David Hasselhoff) wears a Speedo trunk with a fullish fit, while Cody (David Chokachi) fills his slot in a snugger TYR red sport trunk. Off the job, Mitch goes for the aging beach-bum, dune-buggy-dude effect (or should we say affect?), in black or blue boxer-style trunks. Cody, however, strikes a more youthful stance with Hawaiian surf-style shorts and lovely, free-flowing TYR briefs. Thus, the phrase "hang ten."

'Cause Everyone Dresses Down Differently

Man cannot live on odd scraps of Lycra alone (okay, maybe man could, but woman would never allow it). Consequently, even the Baywatched are forced to don over-garments from time to time. Heavy sigh. Still, as aggrievous as these moments might be, they do allow the show's fine troupe of actors to make some creative fashion statements. "Every cast member has unique personality and flair," says Braverman, "and they incorporate their clothing into their characters."

Take C. J.'s flower-child, sex-kitten, do-me-now-hard-and-fast-against-the-lifeguard-chair look. You've got the cutoff jeans with platform shoes, the '70s-style floral shirts in with wide bell-sleeves, the body-hugging knit dresses from Bisou Bisou, the cropped baby Ts with plunging necklines in ice cream colors. Or take her aquatic animal theme (please): the sterling dolphin pendant, the sea lion earrings, the shell ankle bracelets. This is unique personality and flair on some sort of cosmic meta-level. On the other hand, says Braverman, Neely is "the vampish one" (thank God she cleared that up for us). "She's sexy and upscale, a Newport Beach type. Her character has more money than the others, which means she isn't a working girl." So, wait—the others are *working*? Furthermore, "Her character's catlike and plotting," comments Braverman. "To convey this concept, her clothes are slinky, flowy, shiny—lots of silk skirts, clingy knits, dresses with spaghetti straps, and sandals."

Less earthy, more mall-y, Caroline is a Contempo Casuals chick (in real life, mind you, Yasmine Bleeth is a high-fashion *Homo sapiens*). "We're able to use vibrant colors on her like hot pinks and lime greens because she's a brunette," says Braverman. Everything in her closet is formfitting and sleek: baby Ts, halter tops, miniskirts and dresses—although hemlines and necklines don't quite approach C. J.-status. The baubles of choice are beads and pearls, and some small drop necklaces with heart-shaped charms. Older sister Stephanie takes a more grown-up, less frilly route: floral sundresses, jeans, vests, crew-neck Ts, sleeveless mock turtlenecks (to show off those thoroughbred shoulders), and moderately short skirts. Her jewelry consists mainly of pierced studs and small crystal bead necklaces. Quoth Braverman: "Stephanie has a classic, tailored look that's still soft and feminine." Compared to the rest of them, she's practically . . . *bookish.*

On the guy side, Mitch is the resident Blue Boy. More Gaines Burger than Gainsborough, this beefcake wears all shades of blue except navy. Ironic. "We like to accent David's incredible blue eyes," says Braverman, "so we put him in periwinkle, teal, turquoise, and purple polo shirts, sweatshirts, or ribbed Ts. Since he has a thirty-three inch waist and a thirty-six inch inseam, many of his trousers are custom made." (Thus, the phrase, "hang twelve.") Cream linen trousers, pleated pants, and Levi's 501 jeans cover his southern exposures; sneakers or loafers, a woven belt with a silver buckle, nubbly raw silk sport coats, and a leather jacket complete the ensemble. And when the *Baywatch* nights get hot, Mitch struts his stuff in an open vest with no shirt underneath. "He's very buff," says

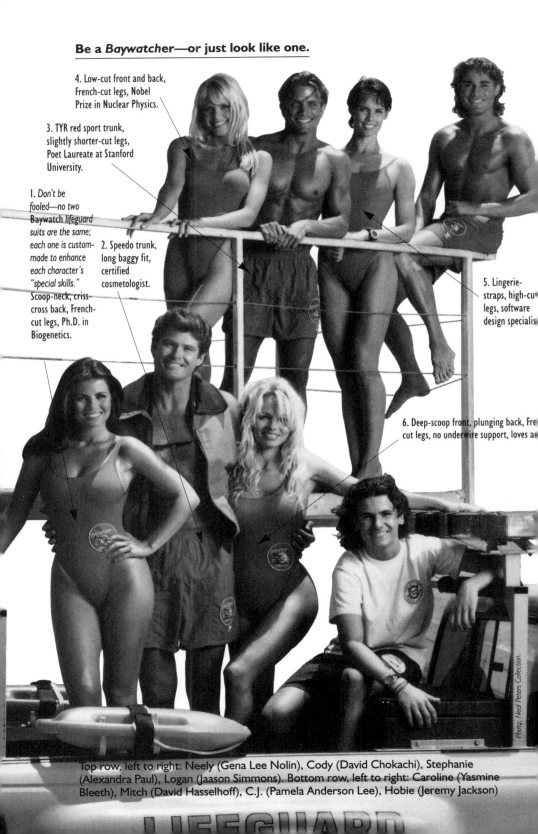

Be a *Baywatcher*—or just look like one.

4. Low-cut front and back, French-cut legs, Nobel Prize in Nuclear Physics.

3. TYR red sport trunk, slightly shorter-cut legs, Poet Laureate at Stanford University.

1. *Don't be fooled—no two Baywatch lifeguard suits are the same; each one is custom-made to enhance each character's "special skills."* Scoop-neck, criss-cross back, French-cut legs, Ph.D. in Biogenetics.

2. Speedo trunk, long baggy fit, certified cosmetologist.

5. Lingerie-straps, high-cut legs, software design specialis

6. Deep-scoop front, plunging back, Fre cut legs, no underwire support, loves a

Photo: Neal Peters Collection.

Top row, left to right: Neely (Gena Lee Nolin), Cody (David Chokachi), Stephanie (Alexandra Paul), Logan (Jaason Simmons). Bottom row, left to right: Caroline (Yasmine Bleeth), Mitch (David Hasselhoff), C.J. (Pamela Anderson Lee), Hobie (Jeremy Jackson)

Braverman. "He works out a lot and likes to show his body." Take it off. Take it all off. Oh, baby. Yeah. Not to be outdone, Cody perpetuates his "bad boy on the beach" reputation in beat-up jeans, earthtone fitted Ts, short-sleeved Hawaiian shirts unbuttoned over T-shirts, and boots. He also sometimes wears Birkenstocks. We guess that would be for his "Christ-boy on the beach" look.

'Cause This Is Reality, Dammit

If you read *Playboy* for the articles, then clearly you tune in to *Baywatch* for the gritty, documentary-style realism. And well you should. "People have no idea what we're dealing with when we shoot the show," says Braverman. "Every day we're fighting the elements." For one thing, it's cold out there. Accordingly, explains Braverman, "When characters fall into the water fully dressed, they need to wear a wet suit underneath to protect them from hypothermia. Since light materials become transparent when wet, I have to find ways to conceal the wet suit—usually with darker colors and sturdier fabrics." They don't call her the queen of Neoprene for nothing. Off camera, Braverman has a vast supply of terry-cloth robes, both long and short, for the cast members to wear while they're waiting to shoot. Incidentally, PAL insists on wearing a short white robe. Sounds real toasty to us.

As if chattering teeth weren't enough to contend with, there's also the continuity issue. Since *Baywatch* isn't shot in sequence, Braverman has to keep track of every article of clothing that hits the sand or brushes the waves. For example, let's say that Mitch spots a drowning child on one of those aforementioned hot *Baywatch* nights. He throws off his vest, dives into the water, rescues the kid, retrieves his vest, and goes on to meet the gang for some disco-fever fun. Now, let's say that the episode-ending disco scene is the first scene shot that week. Braverman has to remember in advance to dust the vest with sand and splash it with salt water prior to Mitch's big "electric slide" finale. Otherwise, it'd be totally unbelievable.

But hold on to your buoys, reality-lovers—there's more! You know the flotation device they carry around? It has this strap? That goes around the body? And when the actors run into the water, they hold it? And when they dive in, they let go? And it's tethered to their waists? That's called a flotation can—*just like the ones real lifeguards use.* And you know what else? That watch on David Hasselhoff's wrist? The one that's waterproof? And tells the time? That's called a lifeguard watch—*and it's just like the real watches that real lifeguards use.* And another thing? You know the lifeguards? When they're at their stations? And how they never wear any jewelry except real lifeguard watches? That's because *real lifeguards never wear jewelry except real lifeguard watches when they're really on duty.*

Yep. This show's the gen-u-ine article.

Baywatch—Accept No Substitutes

Naturally, there are a slew of pretenders—everyone wants a piece of the action. Below, a quick reference guide so you won't be fooled by the competition.

The real thing:

Baywatch—syndicated television show featuring the most current California lifeguard fashions.

Not to be confused with:

Bay Path—junior college in Longmeadow, Massachusetts.

Balkhash—lake in a former republic of the USSR located in Central Asia.

Mayor Koch—(Edward I.) mayor of New York City from 1977 to 1989.

Bobbywach—alleged nickname of Scottish physicist Sir Robert Alexander Watson-Watt (1892–1973).

Bewitched—long-running television sitcom (1965–1973) starring Elizabeth Montgomery as a suburban housewife with extraordinary powers.

Birch Bayh—senator (D) from Indiana.

Gray Swatch—Swiss-made sport timepiece in neutral color.

Gravlax—Swedish cured salmon frequently eaten with pumpernickel toast points.

Spray 'n' Wash—liquid laundry stain remover that fights even the toughest grease stains.

Say what?—popular vernacular meaning "I beg your pardon?"

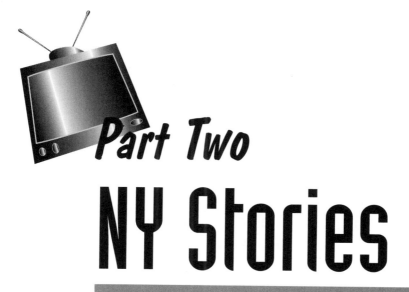

Part Two
NY Stories

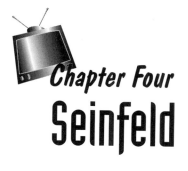

Chapter Four
Seinfeld

THURSDAY, 9:00 P.M. (NBC) SEINFELD

(1989–present). Sharp-edged comedy about four self-absorbed New Yorkers who get in various zany scrapes and live to complain about them. Casual urban styles, hem-and-haw-lines, and seam-splitting perils, all fashioned out of classic Kvetch-22 material. More commotion than emotion, but funny—like a crutch.

Did you ever notice how in Jerry's apartment they're always standing? Eating cereal and standing. Talking on the phone and standing. George loses his job: They stand and talk about it. Elaine's dating a psychotic? She leans on the couch with Jerry and Kramer poised close by. Maybe George makes a little move toward the refrigerator or something, but that's pretty much it. Not that there isn't any action. There's lots of action. They ponder, gesture, grin, even make sudden movements, all while standing. People get held at gunpoint and ingest poison; they yell and run and spit. But in no time, they're back at the apartment, discussing the day's events, and adopting a "ready stance" for the next surprising event that comes down the pike.

What is the deal with all that standing?

Simple. Standing is funny. Sitting: not funny. That's why there's no work for "sit-down comedians." This can be documented in everyday life. Tower of London: funny. Grand Canyon: not funny. Eyebrows are funny. Ankles are not so funny. Even when you get angry, you want a gesture that has some altitude. Sneering is good, but tap dancing rarely intimidates. Somebody cuts you off in traffic? Rarely do you give them "the toe." Besides, sitting down is for guys who need something. If you're sitting down, you're probably saying, "Could I please get some service over here?" or "Bob, I'll have to mull that over." But when you're standing, you've got edge. You can use funny words like "cummerbund," "underpants," and "haberdashery."

Even better, you can wear cummerbunds, underpants, and assorted haberdashery items without getting them wrinkled—and still be funny. An important consideration, since *Seinfeld* is all about getting the laugh. Essentially, you've got a half hour of comics *sans* relief; as such, every stitch of clothing is relentlessly aimed for the humerus. Sure, you might think that Jerry and the gang simply dress to go to the diner, buy fruit, and . . . stand around. You might believe that the clothes are irrelevant, that the dialogue's the key. Ah, so young. So naive. Fact: When you're number one, everything is calculated. Or so we hear. Even George Costanza knows that there's no such thing as a free laugh.

They say the secret to comedy is good timing (or alternatively, good clown shoes!). On *Seinfeld*, they have a few more tricks to trade. Below, four comedy secrets from *Seinfeld*'s closet to get you on the laugh track. And if all else fails, you can always try a little song, a little dance . . . a little seltzer down your pants.

1. You've Gotta Have a Straight Man

The comic concept: By straight, we don't mean heterosexual, although, as it happens, none of the men on *Seinfeld* is gay (not that there's anything wrong with that). In the comedic sense, the straight guy—gay or otherwise—sets up jokes and reacts to others; he deadpans, he smirks, he is the master of his domain. Essentially, when a wisecrack's tossed out, he's the backboard that provides rebound.

The motivation: No straight guy, no laughs. Imagine if Lou Costello stood with a microphone in front of a brick wall and said, "Who's on first? I'll tell you: a gentleman by the name of Who. And what's on second? Well, that would be a certain fine fellow named What." So very not funny. You need a Lewis for every Martin. A pot for every lid. A lid for every eye. An eye for every ball. A Ball for every Arnaz.

Character to watch: Jerry (Seinfeld). What makes *Seinfeld* particularly brilliant is that their straight guy—the setter-upper, the reactor—is himself a stand-up comedian! So the beauty here is that Jerry actually is playing a dual role. Yup. *It's spooky.*

The getup: Crisp and clean, and meta-caffeine.

How to dress the part: It varies, depending on whether Jerry's delivering his monologue or engaging in dialogue. *In medias* riff, his garb has a bit less spit, more polish. "That red curtain behind him drives me nuts," says *Seinfeld*'s costume designer Charmaine Simmons. "Subtle colors disappear against it. I usually put him in blue shirts, a patterned tie, and sport coats from Armani, Canali or Valentino in blue, olive, forest green, or brown." His on-camera/offstage gear is looser: button-down shirts, sweatshirts, barn jackets; on dates, he might throw a vest into the mix. "But you never see Jerry's upper arms," Simmons points out. All the better to hide something up his sleeve. Below the belt, Jerry's a terminal Levi's 501s man—he wears them both on the show, and in real life. And directly at waist level (which really is thirty-two inches, by the way), he straps on leather belts from Coach and Armani. "Jerry goes for a simple, classic look," says Simmons. Nothing shocking or out of the ordinary—perfect straight-man material.

What is the deal with all those: Shoes. For a while, Jerry wore white Nikes and nothing but. Recently, though, he's kicked the habit and moved on to Timberland boots.

Incidentally: Have you ever noticed how men like shoes that denote some activity? Sneakers, loafers, slippers. Work boots, but only on the weekends. To the male mind, shoes are symbolic. They mean something. Women should pay attention to this. For instance, on a first date, pumps are good. They heighten the sexual potential. Spectator pumps? Even better. If the guy's not sure, he might ask. "So, about those shoes of yours, what do you call them, anyway? Mules? Hmm. Interesting." Meanwhile, his brain cells are screaming, "Get out of there! She's wearing mules! Dodge the bullet before it's too late!" Then again, if he's really attracted to her, he may think, "Okay. Not a disaster. Could be clogs."

Laugh with or at: With—after all, he's the one laughing at everyone else. Besides, what kind of twisted person laughs at the straight guy?

2. You've Gotta Move

The comic concept: The art of falling with flair is possibly America's greatest contribution to comedy (and we mean that in the most ironic way possible). It started with a pie in the face, and snowballed to include pratfalls, walking into walls, and in the most sophisticated circles, knees to the groin. Ah, the quiet majesty of testicular humor.

The motivation: As Mel Brooks once said, comedy is when you fall into a manhole; tragedy is when I prick my finger. Why is it funny to watch some numnut (or should we say numb-

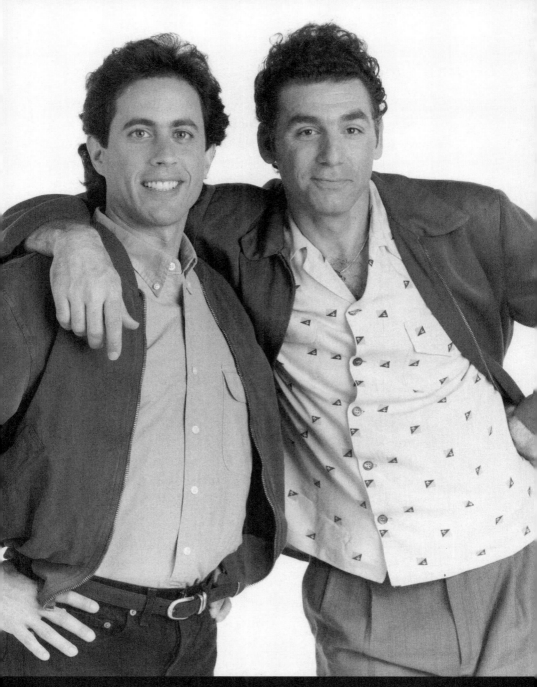

We're number one! We're number one! Dressed to thrill, spill and cavil—
Seinfeld's Jerry (Jerry Seinfeld) and Kramer (Michael Richards) are the two,
the proud, the depraved. With neighbors like that, who needs *Friends*?

nuts?) get his block knocked off? Intellectually, we have no idea. Luckily, intellect has nothing to do with it.

Character to watch: Cosmo Kramer (Michael Richards). The man who gave non-skid threshold strips a whole new meaning.

The getup: Bright colors, baggy clothes, big shoes, red nose—the basic school uniform at Clown College.

How to dress the part: Physical humor requires precision dressing. "Kramer takes so many spills, and makes such crazy entrances and exits, he needs clothes that allow movement," says Simmons. "We have to find fabrics that don't restrict him—rayon and silk work well. Plus, almost all his clothes are vintage style, because Kramer's not the kind of character who wears what everyone else is wearing. He's different." So different, in fact, that many of his pieces are custom-tailored. "Antique pieces are usually made for smaller people," says Simmons. "Michael's not a small guy." Consequently, Simmons goes to swap meets, conventions and antique fabric shows, buys the raw material, and creates the shirts herself. "We have a Kramer pattern; it's a classic vintage prototype. The fabric is always bold, broad stripes, never neat pinstripes. And we make three or four of the same shirt for each show. That way, if he spills something or rips a seam, we have backups." His windmill gait also demands a modicum of legroom, in the form of roomy, shiny trousers that smack of the late fifties. Again, they aren't necessarily bona fide antiques—Simmons often leans on more current vintage knockoffs by designers like Perry Ellis. "If the fabric looks too new," she adds, "it's distressed and washed to look like it could be thirty years old." Doc Marten lace-ups are the toe-stubbers of choice. And for full-moon nights, nothing gets between Kramer and his Calvins.

What is the deal with all those . . . Pants. In addition to the baggy cut, all of Kramer's pants are shortened. "We hem them above the ankle to add to his oddness," explains Simmons.

Incidentally: Why is it that everything above the waist is singular, while everything below the waist is plural? You put on a shirt, a sweater, a jacket. Then move lower down, and suddenly you're wearing pants, shorts, trunks, briefs. Briefs! If they're so brief, how can there be two of them? It's as though your legs merit individual attention, but your arms get lumped into a single entity. Somewhere along the line, all the lower body parts got together and held a meeting: "Look, we've got to get better representation. Remember what happened when Tonsils and Appendix decided to manage themselves? They got removed! It was a disaster! Now, rumor has it that certain areas on this body are about to be downgraded, and it's not going to be us."

Laugh with or at: At, no holds barred. Kramer thrives on ridicule. Hello, sad clown. We know you're in there!

3. You've Gotta Dress for Distress

The comic concept: Whether you're watching Shakespeare or slapstick (or possibly a more reasonable oeuvre in between), you're bound to come across the scapegoat. You'll recognize him instantly: He's the one who drops the ball, loses the girl, or takes the heat—all for the sake of your viewing pleasure.

The motivation: Comedy via errors. If you can't laugh until you cry, cry until they laugh. Added bonus: If you act beleaguered enough, they might even think you're kind of cute. Think Stan Laurel. Charlie Brown. Stimpy. For some reason, it's not a good party until everybody gets to spit at the fat kid.

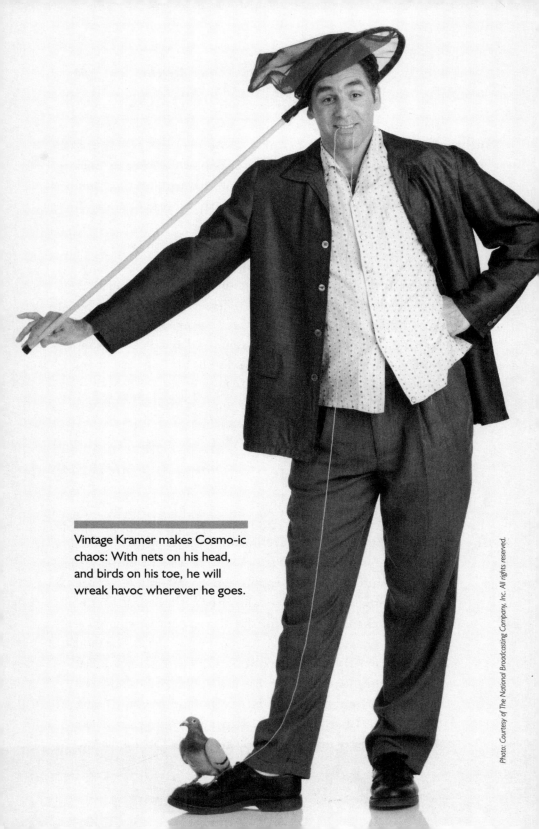

Vintage Kramer makes Cosmo-ic chaos: With nets on his head, and birds on his toe, he will wreak havoc wherever he goes.

Why the universal tendency toward schadenfreude? Ask Sigmundfreude.

Character to watch: George Costanza (Jason Alexander). When he's not getting fired for sleeping with the office cleaning woman, he's being railroaded into organizing a charity foundation in memory of his thankfully deceased fiancée or living miserably with his long-embittered parents who are more concerned with their *TV Guide* collection than their son's dangerously high blood pressure. George can't even cut himself a little slack. The one time he received rave reviews in the bedroom (courtesy of the Risotto Girl), he was convinced she was lying. In retrospect, she probably was.

The getup: Garments that restrict, suffocate, and ensure that he's bound for gags.

How to dress the part: Hot and tight (in a bad sense, not a good one). "George is forever having a hard time, and his clothes convey this—if they're snug, he comes off as even more strung out," says Simmons. This means shirts that pinch at the jugular, ties that circumscribe like a Salem-made noose, and ubiquitous khakis (the same cut in four colors) that strain until the waistband doubles over in surrender. Think shrinkage. "We also like to put George in dorky outfits," says Simmons. "We'll layer him in a sweater or a vest. He's got two trench coats: One's Woody Allenish, the other has epaulets and a huge collar—they're sort of depressing." All a part of his master plan. Now that he's a Yankee, George wears sport coats to the office; away from work, he wears puffy jackets and anoraks that tie him into an unwilling hourglass figure. Any item that's rich in contrast or texture works for George, as long as it gives the impression that he's about to pop.

What is the deal with all those: Ties. George wears more ties than any other person on the show. They're usually wide, dark, and not very expensive. "We see him as the average guy—he might shop at Sears or J. C. Penney," says Simmons. Not that there *are* any Sears or Penneys in Manhattan, but it's the thought that counts.

Incidentally: You have to wonder what was going through the mind of the guy who invented ties. Did he look in the mirror one morning when he was shaving and think, "Mmm . . . not quite right. Close, but something's missing. Maybe if I wound my bathrobe belt around my neck, and tied it into a knot at the base of my throat . . . uh-huh, uh-huh, not bad. Pretty sharp!" And then he stuck on a stray bobby pin so the belt wouldn't hang into the sink, and invented the tie clip, too.

Laugh with or at: In our opinion, laugh at, cry with—but it's your ball game. You make the call.

4. You've Gotta Have Contrast

The comic concept: If sitting is less funny than standing, same is less funny than different. Again, this is easy to document in everyday life. Identical twins: not funny. Mismatched socks: funny. Ann Landers and Dear Abby: not so funny. The Captain and Tennille: very funny. Rarely does a joke begin with, "So a white guy and another white guy are walking down the street . . ." In shoe stores, you hardly ever hear a salesman say, "Hey, Bill, get a load of this. That buffoon over there? You'll never believe—*his feet are exactly the same size!*"

The payoff: With one quick hit of the contrast button, setups become more vivid, punch lines become sharper. In successful ensemble-humor routines, short takes tall, smart takes

57

stupid, the cat takes a mouse, the mouse takes the cheese—
and the cheese, of course, stands alone.

Character to watch: The loveliest limburger of them all, Elaine
Benes (Julia Louis-Dreyfus). In early shows, she wondered
aloud why she was hanging out with such a loser crowd. Six
seasons later, she vowed to break free from the selfsame
loser crowd. This is not to imply that her point of distinc-
tion is winning. No one on *Seinfeld* does a whole lot of winning. Rather, Elaine stands alone because she's, you know, a
chick.

The getup: An extensive wardrobe that makes you pretty enough to
balance out the picture. In this case, Elaine has to be beautifully tailored and put together in such a way that she comes
off as an X-chromosome diamond in the Y-chromosome
rough.

How to dress the part: Elaine's clothing reflects fashion trends far
more than that of her counterparts. "She's gone through
pleated skirts, minis, long skirts," says Simmons. "We keep
everything she wears. Then, when a hemline comes back
into fashion, we reach into her closet and pull it out again—
just like a real person would do. If a lot of action's required,
she wears pants." Her color palette primarily consists of
dark, New Yorky shades of maroon, brown, black; her
designer palette has heavy shadings of Calvin Klein. The silhouette is reminiscent of the forties—broad shoulders, tiny
waist. "We put her in fitted clothes," says Simmons, "so she
looks feminine next to the guys. She wears a lot of jackets—
some long, some short vintage pieces. We tend to mix it up
a lot, especially since she started working for J. Peterman.
It's a progressive company, so she can experiment more."
(F.Y.I.: When we see Elaine sitting at her desk, she's usually
gussied up only above the waist, to save time for the next
costume change.) Furthermore, "Soft romantic sweaters are

great on her. Also, V-necks, because of her beautiful neck and bustline." Evidently, this is the bustline to die for—it led one network TV exec to join Greenpeace and drown trying to save the whales. Finally, Elaine is wont to don a pair of sexy-librarian glasses for extra-hard moments of thought, and a black leather car coat for extra-dangerous capers like, say, dog-napping.

What is the deal with all those: Earrings. Not to mention necklaces. Simmons chooses eclectic, vintage pieces, either purchased from antique stores or custom-designed. "Nothing matches on Elaine; she'll wear little earrings from one place, and a necklace from another. She mixes different stones, and different eras." Which fits in neatly with our contrast theme.

Incidentally: Why do women always want to receive expensive jewelry as gifts? If it's a really nice piece, they can't even wear it. If it's a really, really nice piece, they can't even keep it around. They pay a person at the bank to lock it in a box for them. So some poor guy spends his life savings to buy a diamond bracelet for his wife, and then he has to take out a loan to rent an apartment for it! Where is the pleasure in this? Maybe it's an emotional security thing. Maybe when she goes to the safe deposit, the guard says, "Another shiny, useless rock? What does that bring the total to now, eight? I've gotta tell you, Mary, you are one lucky woman. He must really care."

Laugh with or at: With. She's the token woman in the crowd. If we laughed at her, she could, like, sue.

Not out of the realm of possibility, considering the characters' litigious natures. These people do not take things sitting down (see first paragraph of chapter). They can't afford to—hey, the one character who spent too much time

Be a *Seinfeld*ian—or just look like one.

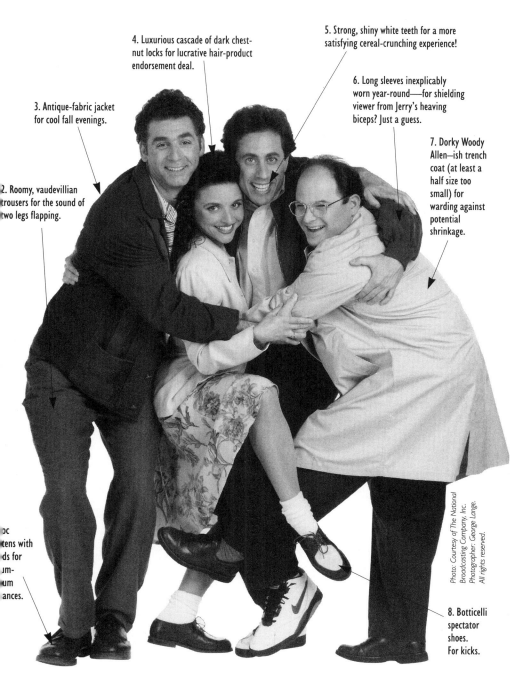

3. Antique-fabric jacket for cool fall evenings.

4. Luxurious cascade of dark chestnut locks for lucrative hair-product endorsement deal.

5. Strong, shiny white teeth for a more satisfying cereal-crunching experience!

6. Long sleeves inexplicably worn year-round—for shielding viewer from Jerry's heaving biceps? Just a guess.

7. Dorky Woody Allen–ish trench coat (at least a half size too small) for warding against potential shrinkage.

2. Roomy, vaudevillian trousers for the sound of two legs flapping.

oc tens with ds for um- um ances.

8. Botticelli spectator shoes. For kicks.

Left to right: Kramer (Michael Richards), Elaine (Julia Louis-Dreyfus), Jerry (Jerry Seinfeld), and George (Jason Alexander) sitting and licking envelopes ended up dead. Still, despite their amusing, subtle vertical pratfalls, or rather, "prat-stands," the one glitch in hanging out with the *Seinfeld* gang is that sooner or later, you can pretty much bet your boots that one of them will somehow get mad at you. They're programmed to get mad at you. They're paid to be mad at you. After a while, it's enough to make you pine for a couple of characters who might be, oh, say, mad *about* you. Well, pine no further. ***Mad About You***—coming up next.

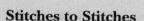

Stitches to Stitches

The writers of *Seinfeld* love to use articles of clothing to drive plot lines. Below, some pivotal pieces of apparel and the stories behind them.

1. The Baked Trench

In which Kramer goes through an episode of wanting to wear his clothes straight from the dryer so they'll be warm and toasty. After getting caught in the rain, Kramer convinces a pizza man to stick his coat into the pizza oven. It gets burned, natch, and frying pan spawns fire in no time flat (okay, make that twenty-two minutes). According to Simmons, "We actually had to use two different coats—before burn and after burn. We couldn't get multiples—it was a one-of-a-kind coat—so we used a lighter shade of coat for the pre-burn scenes. Sometimes you have to take a little comedic license."

2. The Bra that Didn't Fit

In which Kramer sues a woman—actually, the heiress to the Oh Henry candy bar fortune—for walking around in a bra with no top (he claims that her indecent exposure distracted him when he was driving and caused him to crash his car). At the trial, the heiress is asked to try on the bra. It doesn't fit; the judge must acquit. "I custom-made it from off-white lace," remembers Simmons. "Since the actress had to move around in it quite a bit, I based the pattern on a jog bra to be sure it provided enough support."

3. The Bro

In which George sees his father shirtless, and experiences his own personal *Crying Game* shock-epiphany. Consequently, Kramer comes up with the idea of a male pectoral support system—a bra for men that he dubs "the Bro." Simmons designed it herself, using two jock straps. "I had to make it over a weekend. When Jerry Stiller [George's father on the show] wore it for the first time, he put it on backward."

4. The Puffy Shirt

In which Jerry makes a major charity appearance, and unwittingly agrees to wear a shirt designed by Kramer's soft-talking girlfriend. Naturally, Simmons created this garment, too. "I started with an old Laurence Olivier shirt from the Paramount costume warehouse," she says, "and fashioned it into something that was even worse. Jerry then wore it in real life on *The Tonight Show with Jay Leno.*"

5. The Executive

In which Kramer teams up with Jerry's father and markets a line of beltless trench coats to a vintage clothing store. All goes well—until moths intervene. Says Simmons, "I went out, bought the most basic London Fog raincoats, and yanked all the belts off—that was an easy one."

6. Kramer's Jeans

In which Jerry points out that Kramer never wears jeans, and insinuates that this is due to his expanded waistline. To prove he is still lithe and trim, Kramer purchases a pair of skintight, cowboy-fit Wranglers, gets stuck like a fly in amber, and all chaos ensues. In the scene where Kramer flops about like a fish while Jerry attempts to pull the jeans off him, Simmons recounts, "Michael was thrashing around so much, he ended up throwing his back out."

7. Elaine's Botticellis

In which Elaine buys a new pair of shoes that are coveted by all, and spends most of the episode trying to hang on to them. "This show was a classic Larry David story line: find something that's completely nothing and make it huge," says

Simmons. "The shoes themselves weren't particularly spe-cial—I bought them at a department store. They were just classic white-and-black spectator shoes."

8. The Ugliest Dress in the World

In which Elaine goes shopping at Barneys, buys a dress, and experiences the universal shopping phenomenon: Stuff always looks way better in the store than it does at home. Simmons fashioned the offending frock from a black velvet dress by Zelda. "We opened it down the front, and added to the skirt to make it bigger. At first, we also put a bow on the back, but eventually we took it off. The dress was horrible. I never wanted Julia to feel that the dress was too ugly to be funny, so she had a lot of input about it."

9. Jerry's Jacket with the Crest

In which Jerry wants to try a new distinguished look, and buys himself a blazer with a crest on the pocket. Later, hav-ing decided he hates the man who sold it to him, he opts to return the jacket, out of sheer spite. "It was just a normal blue blazer," says Simmons. "We designed the crest with enough color to make it pop."

10. The Black-and-White Dress

In which Jerry meets a woman who's wearing a striking black-and-white dress and asks her out. On their first date, she wears it again. On their second date, Jerry wonders if she even owns another piece of clothing. "We got the script on Friday and when Sunday came along, Jerry inserted a line about Superman, who doesn't change his clothes," says Simmons. "The whole idea of a two-toned Spandex dress with a silly neckline seemed to work with the Superman idea, so we went for it."

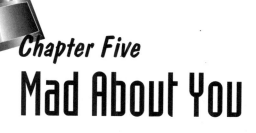

Chapter Five

Mad About You

TUESDAY, 8:00 P.M.(NBC) MAD ABOUT YOU

(1991–present). New York, New York—it's a cuddly town; the mood is up and the comforter's down. The people live in . . . an unbelievably nice apartment. Here the joys and oys of coupledom all wrapped up in snuggly flannel and fleece. Cute characters, cute outfits, cute dilemmas. Cute.

You know the Buchmans, don't you? Talk about a really good life: Jamie has that real great job, and Paul has that real down-to-earth kind of humor, and they have real terrific friends, and they got a really amazing deal on their couch, and their dog is really, really adorable. They're just so *real*.

Except for the pluperfect marriage part. Or the way Jamie gets a big job in a mayoral campaign after just one interview. Or how Paul and Jamie simultaneously contemplate infidelity, teeter on the brink of divorce, squabble in Central Park, take a musical tour of Times Square, weepily reconcile and then, PRESTO!, get pregnant—all in the span of two "very special" episodes. Meanwhile, they're so totally not real. Not even close.

Nonetheless, we'll buy it. We'll buy it because frankly, if it was hard-bitten reality we were after, we'd flip off the TV, wait until 2 a.m., throw on all our jewelry, jump in a wheelchair, and pay a long, fumbling visit to the nearest sidewalk ATM. We'll buy it because amid all the snuggly, soft-focus love, we can still recognize a glimmer of ourselves. Most of all, we'll buy it because we can afford to. Clothes-wise, that is. The dialogue may be scripted, the apartment may be massive, but the clothes are for real. No doubt about it.

No fluke, either. In the big picture, "Believability is the most important factor in deciding how we dress the actors," says Howard Sussman, costumer for the *Mad About You* men. "Of course, budget is a consideration, too, but we always work with the goal of creating a believable character in a realistic setting." Both Sussman and the women's costumer, Audrey Darin, make a concerted effort to sustain a New York state (or at least City) of mind. "The show's taped in Los Angeles," says Darin. "Whenever we feel we're getting a bit California-ish, we pull back and choose a darker-colored, heavier item. Climate is another element—if Jamie is wearing a sleeveless dress in the middle of the winter, you'll never see her go out without first putting on a coat."

On a smaller-picture scale, "We repeat things a lot," says Darin. "These people are on a budget; they can't afford to wear a new outfit every day." She also takes her characters' schedules into account. "When Jamie's caught in a flurry of activity and doesn't have time to iron, we let the clothes go wrinkled." Uh, couldn't Paul do the ironing? Nah—too unrealistic. Adds Sussman, "We're not a trend show; trendy clothes on not-trendy people get you in trouble. We want the audience to relate to the styles. We constantly ask ourselves, Would this character wear that item? For instance, everything in Paul's wardrobe should scream, Independent Filmmaker in New York."

And if they're not screaming that, they're screaming, Tuck me in! or, Hang me up! or, God forbid you should turn the TV off instead of just hitting the mute button when we're having sex! Oh, wait, that's us. Anyway. Sussman and Darin shed such sartorial light on the characters and the actors who play them, they really came alive for us (the characters, that is—Sussman, Darin, and the actors are already very much alive on their own). We felt that we understood them. That we knew them. That we could *be* them. So much so, in fact, that we felt compelled to run with this trove of style insight and spin through a day in the life of Jamie Buchman/Helen Hunt circa 1995. Join us, won't you?

7:30 a.m. Wake to music. Paul (Paul Reiser) is snoring. Pookie-wookie little Paul. Gosh, you're mad about him.

7:35 a.m. Doze to music.

7:40 a.m. Get out of bed. Notice that the waist of your pajama bottoms is twisted around. Wonder if this means you've lost weight. It's possible—in the past couple years, you've already gone from a size eight to a six. Plus, you've been taking those yoga classes. Feel hopeful and happy.

7:42 a.m. Step on scale. Odd. Paul's old flannel shirt must be weighing you down. Step off scale, remove shirt and pajama bottoms, step back on scale. Suddenly feel not so hopeful and happy after all. Goddamit! What the hell is going on—stop and realize how very un-Zen you're being. Breathe in, breathe out. *Ohm mani padme ohm . . . ohm mani padme* oh, Jesus, Murray's drinking out of the toilet again. Speculate whether drinking out of the toilet could be bad for his health. Speculate whether kissing him on the lips after he's been drinking out of the toilet could be bad for your health. Okay, enough speculation. Go to sink and brush teeth. Hum "Copacabana."

8:04 a.m. Dress for work. Let's see, let's see. . . . Open your closet door and marvel over the array of boxy, oversized suits you used to wear. Not to mention the silk blouses that were practically your uniform for a year. What were you thinking? So eighties. Rifle through more current collection of restructured vintage suits: navy, nope, taupe, nope, black, not today, gray, maybe. There's not a lot of color happening here. Make mental note to add some pale blues, pinks, maybe a little red.

8:10 a.m. Realize you're running late and had better reach a decision. Settle on a fitted brown jacket from Barneys with an off-white camisole underneath, and Isaac Mizrahi straight-legged pants. Perfect—stylish but not too trendy. Shiny micro-minis are only for girls who are, like, on TV. Not you. You've got a life to lead.

8:15 a.m. Paul stirs in bed, turns over, and opens one eye to watch you dress. "I'm thinking I feel turned on," he announces. "Really?" you ask. "A little bit," he says. You tell him to keep dreaming. Slip into a pair of Robert Clergerie loafers, and put on some teensy white gold hoop earrings with even teensier diamonds.

8:35 a.m. No time for breakfast. Grab black Zelda overcoat with brown velvet collar. Brief pause to reflect: This coat is the best. You love this coat. You're mad about this coat. Leave for work.

9:14 a.m. Major subway problems, yet you still beat Fran (Leila Kenzle) to the office. Wait 'til she hears you got groped on the train. Giggle into your coffee as you picture her horrified expression. Fran rushes in wearing a short skirt—quick double take: *mint green!*—and a long, fitted jacket by Parallel. How does she walk around in heels like that? Your bad knee could never withstand the punishment. She pulls a chair over to your desk and launches into a story about her latest fight with Mark.

9:42 a.m. Continue talking about fight. What a doozy—they sure were mad about something! You and Paul hardly ever fight like that. Sweet, precious, tiny Paul. Your mind wanders. Boy, you never really noticed what big jewelry Fran wears. You're more of a small-jewelry girl yourself. You interrupt her and ask if you can try on her ring. She tries on yours. You each admire the other's but conclude that you both prefer your own on yourselves. This is why you are friends.

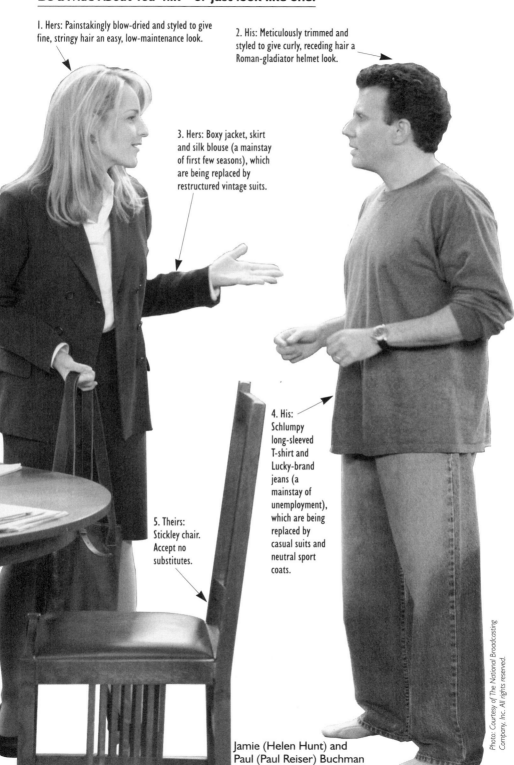

Be a *Mad About You*—nik—or just look like one.

1. Hers: Painstakingly blow-dried and styled to give fine, stringy hair an easy, low-maintenance look.

2. His: Meticulously trimmed and styled to give curly, receding hair a Roman-gladiator helmet look.

3. Hers: Boxy jacket, skirt and silk blouse (a mainstay of first few seasons), which are being replaced by restructured vintage suits.

4. His: Schlumpy long-sleeved T-shirt and Lucky-brand jeans (a mainstay of unemployment), which are being replaced by casual suits and neutral sport coats.

5. Theirs: Stickley chair. Accept no substitutes.

Jamie (Helen Hunt) and Paul (Paul Reiser) Buchman

10:00 a.m. Fran wraps up incredibly long story and gestures dramatically. You can't help but admire her breasts. She complains that they prevent her from wearing cropped jackets, but big deal. Were it an option, you'd make the sacrifice. Make mental note to try on Wonderbra at Saks.

11:40 a.m. Phone rings. Paul. He's contemplating the eagles on the Chrysler Building again, hoping to reconcile with Yoko Ono. You mention that when you were ordering your basketball sneakers from J. Crew, you saw a leather car-coat on sale just like his, except brown. Possible birthday present? He points out he doesn't wear clothes from catalogs. "I'm thinking you could be more flexible," you remark. "Really?" he asks. "A little bit," you answer.

12:15 p.m. Meet Lisa (Anne Ramsay) for lunch at the department store where she works. She's still in a huff about not being allowed to wear her favorite ripped jeans on the job. You try to be your usual sympathetic self, but come on. How bad can it be? She's pushing the limits of casual chic as is, what with all that mismatched thrift store stuff, and tied-up shirts, and the irrational way she insists on wearing loafers without socks. It's January, for Chrissake. She claims her black cigarette pants keep her ankles warm. Whatever. For the zillionth time, you urge her to buy a skirt. For the zillionth time, she states her refusal to show her legs. It's a little hard to get over. You jokingly inquire whether she wears a special pair of paper pants at the gynecologist. She is not amused.

1:45 p.m. Screw the subway; easier to cab back to the office. During the ride, you muse over the innumerable woman-hours your sister and best friend suck out of your day—the constant calls, the endless tales of woe, the unannounced visits. Ridiculous. It's like they're characters on a sitcom or something. Honestly. Discover to your dismay that you've shut the bottom of your beloved coat in the taxi door, and it's been dragging through the slush for twelve city blocks. *Ohm* like crazy.

2:10 p.m. Give up trying to scrub the grime off your coat. It needs professional help. Hey—just like Lisa and Fran! Your own wit cheers you up considerably. *C'est la vie.* Make mental note to take coat to the cleaners when you pick up Paul's Armani tux.

3:05 p.m. Your boss, Lance, unexpectedly drops by your office to discuss campaign strategy. Wish he'd warned you he was coming; you would've worn a more corporate-looking skirt. You put on your glasses to appear more serious and pretend you're happy to see him. He pretends to believe you.

4:20 p.m. Alone at last. Lift nose from grindstone to soft-focus on Paul. Darling, adorable Paul. Pause a few seconds for a wide private smile.

6:00 p.m. Home again. Paul's in the kitchen, wearing his usual Lucky-brand jeans and a black T-shirt with a denim shirt over it. No vest. Good. The vest look was getting tired on him. Ever since he won that Silver Sprocket award, he's cleaned up his act. He even bought a few casual suits and sport jackets, mostly dark neutrals like charcoal, brown, and navy. He says the guy at Bloomingdale's claims that brown is the new black. *Vogue* says navy is the new brown. So what does that make black—the new blue? This fashion business gets weirder all the time.

6:50 p.m. Remind Paul that you're meeting the guys for dinner. Instruct him (lovingly) to put on navy crepe trousers, that great new orange rayon shirt, and his Barneys blazer. Or else the wool jacket he got at Macy's. Also he should remember to return the Banana Republic striped cardigan shirt he borrowed from Ira. You comment how everyone and their brother has that shirt. "What do you mean?" he says. "Ira's my cousin." Dear, funny, literal Paul.

7:35 p.m. Right before leaving, try out the positive-reinforcement

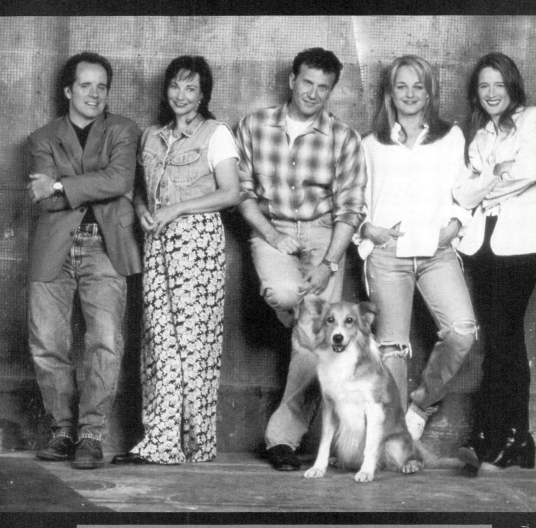

Wardrobes may alter, hairlines may recede, but they'll always be mad about each other. The mainstays of *Mad About You*, starting from the loveable schlub on the left: Cousin Ira (John Pankow) is sporting in a jacket; Fran (Leila Kenzle) goes floral; Paul (Paul Reiser) takes a cotton to casual comfort; Jamie (Helen Hunt, pre–Emmy Award) takes in the hole scene; and Lisa (Anne Ramsay) is stylishly slack. And up front, Murray (Maui the dog) is all glamor in his customary sable and white fur coat.

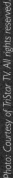

behavior modification you read about in *Cosmo*. Gush to Paul over how much you adore his Armani suede loafers, how manly they make him look, how attracted you are to them. In short, you're mad about those loafers! He wears Nikes anyway. Make mental note to cancel subscription to *Cosmo*.

8:00 p.m. Ira (John Pankow) is late. While you're waiting for him, Mark drones on about the latest fight he had with Fran. Been there, heard that. His wardrobe is as unoriginal as his conversation. The same Calvin Klein suit. Over and over. The polo shirt. The patterned tie. The wingtips. Everything about him screams Established Doctor in New York. It's as if he has a full-time costume person dressing him every morning. Please.

9:02 p.m. Ira finally makes his customary schlumpy appearance— black jeans, Banana Republic bowling shirt, Doc Martens. Not a man who cares about clothes. In the interim, all sorts of cuckoo-nutty things have happened. The ditzy waitress mixed up the orders, brought you another table's food, the other table stormed out, and you ended up having to pay for everything. It's madness, you exclaim aloud, sheer madness! When the antics subside, Ira explains his lateness with a tragicomic tale of seduction and betrayal. Holy smokes. You can't make this stuff up.

11:00 p.m. Bedtime. You and Paul climb into bed. He's changed into a white T-shirt and boxers, and smells Downy fresh. You throw on one of his pajama tops, no bottoms—you're not gonna be rooked by that whole twisted waistband business again tomorrow morning, that's for sure. Paul makes a bunch of ooh-ah-mmph snuggly noises against your shoulder. "I'm thinking I feel turned on," he says. "Really?" you ask. "Very much," he says. You kiss and coo like two doves in a cote, and then Paul does a variety of interesting things to you that would drive a network censor board crazy. He really knows how to hit your V-chip.

11:07 p.m. Watch *Seinfeld* rerun. Paul starts snoring. Pookie-wookie little Paul. Have you mentioned that you're simply mad about him? Your stomach gurgles contentedly; dinner was yummy. The ditzy waitress's mistake turned out to be a good thing after all. Come to think of it, that ditzy waitress kind of reminds you of someone. Barbara Eden? Close, but not quite. The girl from your Vassar freshman English class? Nah—she had dark brown hair. Oh, wait, maybe it's the blonde on that TV show with the great clothes—what's it called again? Something about *Friend*ship, or drinking coffee with your *Friends*, or getting all dressed up to hang out with your *Friends*. Whatever—you're too tired to remember. Make mental note to turn to **Chapter Six.**

Mad to Order

With its wide-ranging closet and universal appeal, *Mad About You* has the potential to spawn any number of stylish spin-offs. An advance look at some future prospects:

Mad About You Magazine

Satirical monthly that lampoons "The Lighter Side of Coupledum." Regular features include Spy + Spy 4-ever, as well as wry mascot Alfred E. Buchman and his catchphrase: "What, me? Rogaine?"

Mad About You Max

Romantic comedy set in the desolate future. Top independent filmmaker Max Buchman is on the verge of retirement, but when crotchety landlord refuses wife, Sadie, permission to install new walk-in closet, Buchman embarks on high-film-speed revenge.

Mad About You Max 2

Max, now a sales representative for the California Closet Company, reluctantly helps tiny SoHo boutique defend itself from obliteration by giant mass-produced-clothing store chain. Not as original as the first, but incredible automatic tie-rack stunts and compelling visual design make it worthwhile. Later renamed *The Clothes Warrior* for Australian release.

Mad About You Max Beyond Underdome

Max, in his third career as a lingerie designer, stumbles upon unethical band of plastic surgeons in remote area of Silicon Valley. Urged on by Sadie, he survives a battle to the death in Roman-style haircut. Lots of action and stunts, but lacks overall support.

Mad About You Cow Disease

Fatally ugly disease in which couples who accrue too

many leather goods find themselves spontaneously singing "I'll Be Loving Moo" in the shower, purchasing Holstein patterned sofas, naming their children "Elsie" or "Bossy," and uncontrollably grazing on Ben and Jerry's.

Mad About You Dog and Glory

Nerdy independent filmmaker (Paul Reiser) makes a large campaign contribution to New York politician (guest star George Pataki), and is repaid by having Helen Hunt delivered to him as a "token of appreciation." They fall in love, get married, acquire a dog, and glory in their utter happiness.

Mad About U2: Rattle and Hum

Scattershot documentary-style video recording the birth of Paul and Jamie Buchman's first baby.

M * A * D About You

Trials and tribulations of Dr. Mark Debanow (Richard Kind), a prominent gynecologist in New York who wears Calvin Klein scrubs and week after week discovers anew that love is a battlefield.

It's a Mad About You, Mad About You, Mad About You, Mad About You World

Sprawling "mad"-cap comedy about a group of New Yorkers, led by Paul and Jamie Buchman, scrambling to find $250,000 Banana Republic gift certificate hidden under office building of *W* magazine. Watch for cameos by Bea Arthur, Gabe Kaplan, David Doyle, Bonnie Franklin and a host of other comedy greats.

Chapter Six
Friends

THURSDAY, 9:00 P.M. (NBC) FRIENDS

(1994–present). Seminal television fashion show, complete with cappuccino, clever repartee, and attitude. Six fabulous bods, six product-driven coifs, six distinct looks, six escalating salaries. With six you get payroll.

11:58 P.M.

Phooey. You've been tossing and turning for hours; what time is it anyway? You check the clock: 11:59. Jeez. Who would've thought the night was gonna be this way? It's not a joke, you know—tomorrow you'll be D.O.A. It's like your brain is stuck in second gear. You start to stress about your day, your week, your month, and even your—okay, stop. You give yourself a shake. If you can't sleep, you can't sleep. Not a big deal. You'll do something productive instead. Like . . . you could read that book your sister lent you, *Snow Falling on Some Sort of Cedar Thingamajigs*. You've really been meaning to do more reading. This could be the dawn of a more literary you! Cool. You close your eyes for a minute to contemplate the prospect. You'll be spouting witty prose like Dick Cavett at cocktail parties . . . sprinkling pithy observations while

you're standing at the punch bowl . . . spouting and sprinkling . . . spinkling and sprouting . . . you're sinkling . . .
zzz . . . you're drowsling . . . zzzzz. . . .

TWANG! Loud guitar strum. You're standing in the middle of a
field. It's night. Six shadowy figures cavort around a giant punch
bowl spouting colored streams of water. They're so dark. So real.
They make you think of Rembrandts. Loud music fills the air; you
hear voices singing:

So someone zipped us into closet fantasy (clap, clap, clap, clap),
And launched a retail line: To dress Must See TV;
It's like a whole new brand of watch-and-wear,
So hem your skirts and crop your shirts, drop fifteen pounds,
     and blow out your hair, 'cause—
They'll be there for you (when your hips need a hug),
They'll be there for you (when your hair needs a plug),
They'll be there for you—and you'll pay for it, too.

Catchy. You're quietly humming along, when the humanoids
notice you; they grab you, they pick you up, *they're going to throw you
into the punch bowl!* SPLASH! they line up and dance wildly, GASP! they
furiously stamp their feet while you struggle to the surface, TWANG,
TWANG, TWANG! the music blares relentlessly, as the biggest
humanoid moves ominously in your direction like a slow-motion
locomotive train. You frantically swim toward a tiny couch and lamp
glowing in the distance—*it's your only hope*—but the humanoid's
gaining on you! He's coming closer, his face is getting longer, he's
right on top of you, he's putting his arms around you, he's—hey,
what's Dick Cavett doing here floatii g around in an inner tube?—
God have mercy, he's *hugging you to death,* and you can hardly
breathe, when suddenly, somecne turns out the light, and he lets
go, and you're falling, you're falling, AAAAAAGHHHHHH. . . .

Shhh, shhh, relax. It was only a dream. You needn't be scared—you're among *Friends*. The most famous friends in the world. If you'd stayed asleep long enough, odds are everything would have been neatly, sweetly resolved, you would've all had a good laugh about your little "punch-bowl misunderstanding," and then you'd give each other pedicures. Because that's the essence of *Friends*: pretty (clothes), painted (apartments), polished (bodies), happy, shiny fantasy. Even the cast members are probably pinching themselves to make sure they're awake. Who could've guessed that this ragtag bunch of incredibly beautiful people would become a national phenomenon (doesn't NBC stand for Nothing But Coincidence)? Nonetheless, the show's style has so permeated our air- and brain-waves, many fans can't stop playing dress-up, even in their sleep. Below, a night gallery of viewers' dreams, culled from colleagues, pals, family, and on-line volunteers. We'll let each subject tell his or her story, give our take on the stream of subconsciousness, and then turn to *Friends*'s costume designer Debra McGuire for some reality-based interpretation. Forget Jung—this is the stuff that Nielsen ratings are made from.

CARRIE, 27

The dream: I'm standing at the top of a fluffy mountain in a long white dress. For some reason, I'm holding a pink princess phone. It rings, and this guy standing next to me in a tux reaches to answer it. When he opens his mouth to talk, he shows these horrible metal teeth. I try to run, but my feet are stuck in some gooey white stuff. Suddenly, I realize—I'm a bride on a wedding cake! I scream, jump out of my shoes, slip on the icing, and tumble down, tier after tier, until I hit my head on an edible flower and black out. When I come to, I'm a policewoman in New York City, writing tickets for illegally parked cars. As I continue down the block, my uniform gradually changes and loosens up, until it's just like some really great outfit. I take off my hat, and my hair has more layers than the wedding cake. I check it out in a rearview mirror. It looks pretty good. I shake my head, write a few more tickets, and I'm walking by a sidewalk cafe when I notice the weirdest thing: Every woman has the exact same haircut as me! I spin around and glance across the street—now every guy has the same haircut as me! I freak out and run into oncoming traffic; a horn blasts in my ear and keeps blasting until I wake up and find out it's really my alarm.

The stream: Clearly, Carrie has a Rachel (Jennifer Aniston) fixation. Just like Rachel, she finds herself stuck in a wedding situation that she's not happy with. The pink princess phone symbolizes the entitlement of her childhood; the groom with metal teeth who answers the phone represents her orthodontist-fiancé, Barry, who always tries to talk and think for her. She breaks free, runs away, and takes a low-paying job that requires a uniform. The fact that she's a policewoman may signify an attempt to bring order to her out-of-control life. That, or she just likes to wear black all the time.

The scheme: A classic case of closet character development. In the first season, says McGuire, Rachel dressed much more the Long Island princess part, "but she went on to have a job that made very little money, and kept a lot of personal integrity—a true princess wouldn't do that." Accordingly, after falling off the wedding cake and hitting the self-discovery track, much of the "couture-y, princess-y" stuff fell by the wayside—expensive Chanel-style suits were usurped by baby Ts, ribbed tanks, and flannel drawstring pants. "In early shows, I wanted it to be clear that these were clothes that she had either borrowed, or that were from her old closet," explains McGuire. "Then, as she was finding out who she was, we slowly replaced them." In terms of Rachel's waitressing gear at Central Perk, the original concept—a denim shirt and black skirt—gradually morphed into more creative outfits. "Originally, [the show's creators] were strict about keeping her in a uniform," says McGuire. "By the second season, I thought, 'I've got to put her in different things.' I stretched it as far as I could, and began designing her coffee shop clothes. I was careful to make them look like she could've found them in a thrift shop." She points out, though, that Rachel's clothes don't necessarily appear old or vintage, just different and unique. Like the policewoman in Carrie's dream, Rachel does wear a lot of black, but mixes it with blues, greens, and browns. Her silhouette is sexy and shapely: Gaultier stretch pants, A-line minis, halter-top dresses, Nic Janik shirts, heeled sandals, and sneakers. As for the hair, McGuire had nothing to do with it.

MICHAEL, 29

The dream: I'm in a desert with grasslands, maybe the Serengeti. I spot a small tribe of Neanderthals standing by some trees, about a mile away. I take a step, and they're right in front of me. The tallest one is hanging his head like a puppy; although he's several inches taller, he has the ability to look up at me. He's wearing a bright red loincloth covered with hearts and holding a small leather bag in his hand. I blink, and he's wearing a crown, holding a trophy in his hand. I blink again, and he's wearing a tweed jacket, holding a rock in his hand. He scratches his head, and opens his mouth to speak. I'm not sure I'll be able to understand his language, but then he says, "Could you *be* any more confused?" I have no idea what he's talking about, and I answer, "No, I couldn't." Then he squirts me with a juice box and kisses me hard on the lips.

The stream: Michael seems to have a Ross (David Schwimmer) complex: He feels slightly removed from the tribe (Ross lives

Prime Cut: The Many Layers of Rachel

What makes this woman unforgettable? Her deeply philo-
sophical bent? Her thirst for knowledge? Her natural button
nose or her sense of adventure or her indomitable spirit in
the face of—CUT! What Makes This Woman Unforgettable:
Take 2. CUT! Take 3? CUT! No matter how many takes we do,
the conclusion will always be the same: HAIRSTYLE!

Mind you, we really like Rachel's haircut. One of us—we
won't name names, but it wasn't Val—actually got Rachel's
haircut. Maybe some of you even tried out Rachel's haircut
(in which case, hey, nice haircut!). It became such the rage
that Jennifer Aniston publicly complained about everyone
having "her" hair. Hello! Earth to Jennifer! First of all, like you
stood at the mirror and cut it yourself? Second of all, ever
hear of a little movie called *Klute,* starring some third-rate
hack named Jane Fonda? She had an awful familiar haircut,
didn't she, Jennifer? Or does the name Farrah Fawcett ring
any bells? Sure, her hair was longer and feathered, but trim
that baby to the shoulders, blow it under and *oh my God, it's
Jennifer Aniston!* Or how about salon giant John Sahag, who
invented the shag twenty-five years ago? Did you even have
hair then, Jennifer? *Did you?* Not to mention Goldie Hawn,
Victoria Principal, or Sammy Jo on *Dynasty.* While we're at it,
Bee Gees much? Frankly, if David Cassidy never got pointed in
the direction of Albuquerque and missed three hair appoint-
ments, he could wear a cute, frilly apron and serve coffee in
great big cups, too! Granted, the layers in the seventies started
higher than yours, but layers is layers, sister, no matter how
you slice 'em. So, not to rain on your innovation parade, *Jen,*
but we figured you ought to know. By the by—if you happen
to see Pamela Anderson Lee, you might clue her in to the fact
that her haircut in *Barb Wire* was a dead ringer for Jane
Fonda's in *Barbarella.* It could save her a lot of embarrassment.

Be a *Friend*—or just look like one.

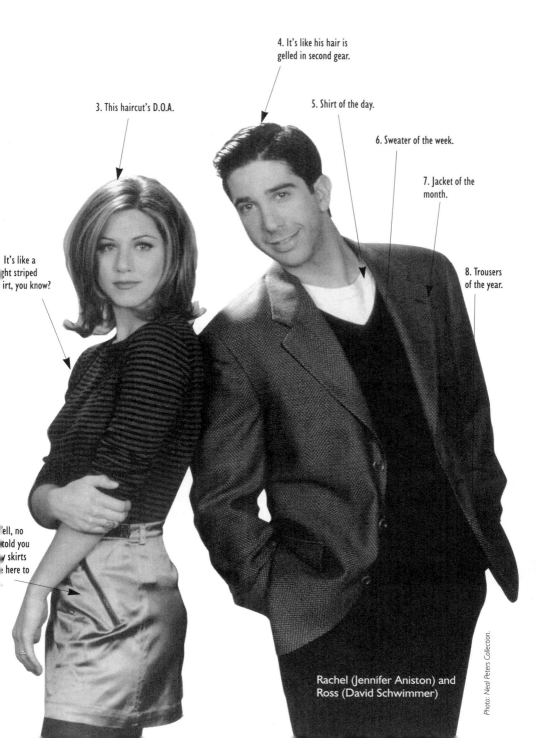

3. This haircut's D.O.A.

4. It's like his hair is gelled in second gear.

5. Shirt of the day.

6. Sweater of the week.

7. Jacket of the month.

8. Trousers of the year.

It's like a
ght striped
irt, you know?

ell, no
told you
skirts
here to

Rachel (Jennifer Aniston) and
Ross (David Schwimmer)

alone, away from the main *Friends* port), and he's befuddled by the constantly changing events around him. Similar to paramour Rachel, Ross is the prince of his family, as evidenced by the crown and trophy. He's also an intellectual paleontologist (tweed jacket, rock), and a not-quite-perfect-fit lover (loincloth/bathrobe borrowed from Rachel, small leather bag/condom). Most of all, though, he means well, *he really means so well.* To this end, he makes an effort to nourish and refresh (squirting juice box), and find love wherever he goes (hard kiss on the lips). That, or he's Ocean Spray's new gay spokesperson.

The scheme: Jack of all trades, master of some. The challenge with Ross is that he plays so many roles in an already crowded cast—responsible brother, world-weary scientist, irresistible boyfriend, dependable pal—and he has to dress for each and every part. The theory of relativity (Monica is his little sister) is subliminally perpetuated by Ross and Monica's parallel palettes. "Their coloring is similar," says McGuire, "I always keep their clothes in the same realm—they're the only two characters who are aligned." Among the males, he's the most colorful of the lot, often sporting vivid shades of blues, greens, and reds. "I could see him wearing a purple turtleneck," says McGuire. "I like to throw a curveball into his character: He can wear a chartreuse shirt under a suit. And I can even use pink on him, although I off-balance it with navy or black." For his museum job, he's professional, but not overly corporate—"the hip end of J. Crew"—in four-button suits, jackets, and flat-front pants designed by Paul Smith, Calvin Klein, and McGuire herself (the suit he wore to ex-wife Carol's wedding was a McGuire original). Interestingly, colleges across the country have reported a recent rise in the number of paleontology majors. Could this *be* a coincidence?

SHARON, 26

The dream: I'm in a room that resembles the inside of a kaleido-
scope—it's full of various colors and shapes. The little
round window is covered with frost; it's snowing like crazy
outside, but I don't feel the cold. Someone hands me a kiwi
smoothie. I look up, and it's a woman in a red shirt wearing
a marshmallow on her head. She says something that
sounds like "Shoes on Kevin Costner." When I don't
respond, she repeats it with increasing agitation until I realize she's saying, "Use a goddamn coaster!" I put my glass on
a magazine; she's not appeased, and maniacally rummages
for a real coaster. I'm beginning to suspect she's crazy, so I
walk to the door. There's a gold hoop hanging on the
door—Marshmallow Head tells me I'm not allowed to leave
unless I jump through the hoop. She jumps through it several times to show me how easy it is, but I know I'll never fit
through that tiny hole. I'd hate her skinny guts, except she
smiles cheerily, and offers to help me exercise and lose
weight. We're jogging in place when a bat wearing a pair of
sunglasses swoops by—I hop on its back and we fly out the
window.

The stream: Many dream analysts claim that living rooms symbolize
the dreamer's psyche—and it just so happens that Sharon's
psyche looks an awful lot like Monica's (Courteney Cox)
West Village apartment. The marshmallow on the woman's
head stands for Monica's toque (that would be the tall white
hat that chefs wear); the bright colors signify Monica's need
to create warmth in a cold, cruel world. Sharon may have a
burning desire to be more ambitious, and the Monica side
of her personality pushes her to achieve. But she resents
being forced to perform (jumping through hoops), and
fears that all her efforts might prove futile (jogging in
place). Finally, the bat is emblematic of the small, secret

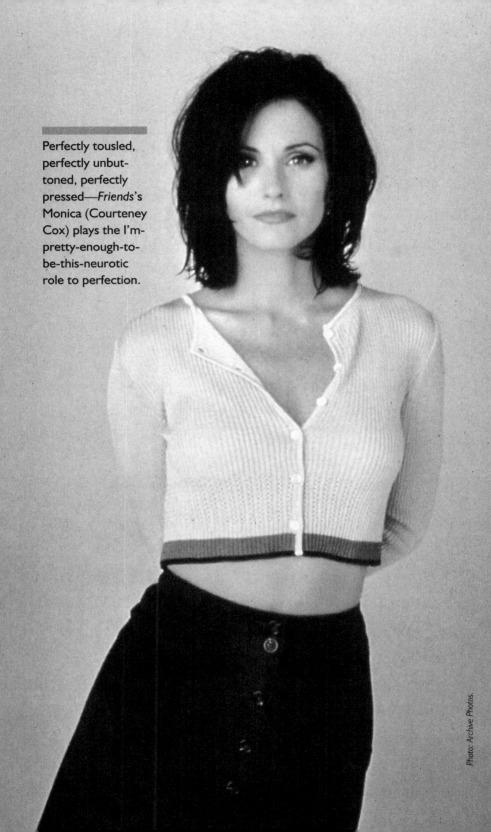

Perfectly tousled,
perfectly unbut-
toned, perfectly
pressed—*Friends*'s
Monica (Courteney
Cox) plays the I'm-
pretty-enough-to-
be-this-neurotic
role to perfection.

Photo: Archive Photos.

wild part of herself that she ultimately would like to surrender to. That, or she has a secret thing for Courteney Cox's ex-Batman, Michael Keaton.

The scheme: Art exemplifies life. As a former painter, McGuire deals with the overall picture as if it were a canvas: "I basically design by palette—and to a certain extent, texture—and go backward from there," she says. "Our sets are so rich in pattern and texture, I need to use a lot of solids for the characters to stand out." Monica, the character who logs in the most time puttering around the biggest, purplest two-bedroom apartment in New York, dresses almost exclusively in deep solids: reds, burgundies, grays and blacks, in the form of A-line dresses, fitted suits, short skirts, and vintage jackets by designers like Nicole Miller, Chaiken & Capone, and Escada. In keeping with her coaster-obsessed personality, she is relentlessly neat, groomed, and clean as a skinny, skinny whistle. To be sure, after she got fired from her job, Monica's look relaxed slightly. "She wears jeans more when she's unemployed, but I usually don't believe in anyone wearing jeans during the work week," asserts McGuire. "I know when I lived in New York, my friends didn't wear jeans to the office."

In addition, on *Friends*, the outfits tend to complement rather than contrast with each other—unlike other costume designers, McGuire is not militant about using different colors on different characters. For instance, at Rachel's surprise birthday party, all three women wore green dresses. "I approached it like I was painting," remarks McGuire. "If I'd been painting three women in a room, I would've dressed them in different shades of green. Plus, if I recall, it was a springtime show, and the green conveyed that the seasons had changed." Which brings up the controversial climate issue: Why do the characters dress summery, even when it's wintery? "I certainly take the weather into account," responds McGuire, "but it's not a primary consideration. Besides, when you're indoors in New York, the heat is overwhelming—people wear less inside there than they do in Los Angeles. It's like the way people don't carry umbrellas in Seattle—that's how they can tell who the tourists are. So it's a question of actual reality versus perceived reality." Mental note to selves: Pack waterproof mascara for next trip to Seattle.

TRISTAN, 31

The dream: I'm standing in an ATM vestibule. There's something screwy with my balance, and I'm going over my past transactions to figure out the problem. Someone comes in; when I glance over, I see that it's Jill Goodacre, the Victoria's Secret model. I'm like, wow! We strike up a conversation, and as we chat, something strange happens: *She starts to grow.* I think I'm imagining it, but no, she's definitely getting bigger— unfortunately, her clothes get bigger too, so I don't get to see any of her naked. From where I'm standing, her head looks enormous. Huge. It has its own satellites. She's blocking the exit, so I try to pretend nothing's wrong and keep talking. The funny thing is, we really get along, and I find myself wondering, if I invite her to my place, will she fit in my apartment? When I finally muster up the courage to ask her, she suddenly shrinks into a little mouse and squeaks, "Oh my gawd! Oh . . . my . . . gawd!"

The stream: Tristan's dream is indicative of acute Chandler (Matthew Perry) Syndrome. Despite his highly controlled environment (an ATM vestibule), he doesn't feel entirely surefooted ("my balance is screwy"), and he needs to review his past transactions (i.e., actions) before he can move on. For Chandler, nothing is perfect or easy—given enough time for scrutiny, even the most exquisite supermodel can develop glaring flaws. The concept of romantic commitment is way too colossal for him to handle; when he does take a step in that direction, he's immediately reminded of old mistakes (in this case, ex-ex-Ohmygawd-girlfriend, Janice). Plainly, Tristan relates to Chandler because they both share a reluctance to grow up and get involved. That, or because they both have funny names.

The scheme: Two steps forward, one step back. If Ross is the character who assumes the most identities, Chandler is the one most trying to find his. Although he makes a concerted effort to move forward (he gets promoted, he feverishly searches for new women), he's also constantly backtracking (he goes back to living with Joey, he revives old flames). And his clothes reflect the emotional flip-flop: One second he's slick and corporate, the next second he's retro. In the morning he's an adult; by evening, he's a tousled little boy. For instance, Big Chandler is wont to wear snappy suits in assorted neutrals like grays or blues; in concordance with his personality, his ties are witty, but rarely astonishing. Still, while he's professional, McGuire points out, "He's not conservative. None of the characters are conservative." Heaven forbid. Little Chandler, on the other hand, messes around in the lightest shade of denim, and rumpled layers of cotton T-shirts, sweatshirts, and sweatpants. Big Chandler favors current high-end designers like Calvin Klein and Hugo Boss. Little Chandler takes a wistful look at the past in retro-style shirts or old standards from Banana Republic, GAP, and J. Crew. "The first year, I made all of Matthew Perry's shirts to give him an unusual retro look," says McGuire, "but then manufacturers began selling the same sort of stuff. When it became too available in the stores, I stopped using it so much." To complete the bifurcated focus, he has two bathrobes: one in navy and green plaid flannel, the other in black and white. In light of this, our razor-sharp fashion sense would lead us to conclude that *plaid flannel works on boys of all ages!*

MICHELLE, 24

The dream: I'm with a bunch of people, sitting by a beautiful brook. It's hot, and I want to jump in, but no one else thinks it's a good idea. I look up at the sky and I can see clouds shaped like birds and flowers. One grayish cloud resembles a cat; another resembles a man I'm vaguely familiar with, but it breaks apart before I can remember who. The sun is beating down, and I'm getting restless and itchy—I can't sit still any longer. So I stand up and dive into the brook. The water is delicious and soothing, and it carries me to exotic and interesting lands.

The stream: Michelle appears to have a strong association with Phoebe (Lisa Kudrow), embracing her sense of whimsy, her strange imagination, and her desire to jump headfirst into life. Birds and flowers represent her idealistic nature, the gray feline-shaped cloud is undoubtedly a "Smelly Cat" metaphor, and the dissolving image of a familiar man could represent Phoebe's thwarted attempts to locate her birth father. Yet despite various hardships—be they chicken pox or lost Ice Capades lovers—Phoebe persists in swimming ahead, and exhibits a Zen-like ability to float wherever the current may take her. That, or she has a terrible sense of direction.

The scheme: Dare to be different—go with the flow. As the token visual wild card, Phoebe is by far the most experimental dresser on the show. She's the girl most likely to wear prints and bright synthetic fabrics—kind of like the cast of *90210* all rolled into one tall blonde. "Phoebe is my

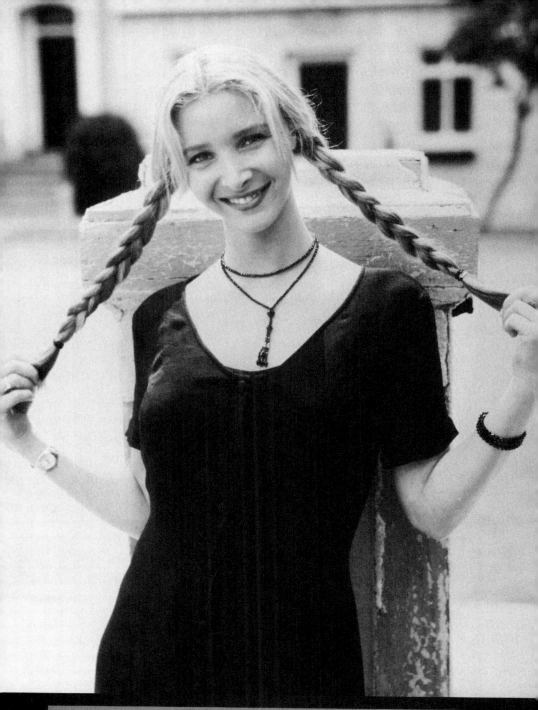

Friends's Pippi, we mean, Hippie, we mean, Phoebe (Lisa Kudrow, we mean Lisa Kudrow, we mean Lisa Kudrow) smiles and holds her hair. We hear this sixties/nineties girl," says McGuire. "I put her in floaty things like bell-bottoms; long, flowing skirts and dresses—she gives me a chance to do a completely different silhouette." This hippie chick's a panoply of patterns: sheer tops with daisy appliqués, Mona Lisa silk-screened jackets, the polka-dot bell-bottom outfit that was green on one side, lavender on the other. Her jewelry is equally eclectic: long beads, giant silver flowers, and dangly earrings, with rings on every finger, and you'd almost swear bells on every toe. McGuire designs a large portion of Phoebe's wardrobe to ensure that "her humor and sensibility will show through." It's like having a visible panty line, but better.

TOM, 26

The dream: I'm walking down the street on a clear, cool day. I'm holding a white lab coat, and somewhere along the way, I drop it. I have a moment of concern, but it passes—I'm feeling confident and carefree, on top of the world. Everything's going great, until I accidentally bump into a guy, and he pushes me down a manhole. As I'm falling, I have an incredibly profound thought, but then I forget what it was.

The stream: Tom's dream has strong Joey (Matt LeBlanc) undertones: It's strong, simple, brief, and brimming with good looks and no-brainer confidence. The dropped white lab coat denotes Joey's brief stint as a doctor on *The Days of Our Lives*, the fall down the manhole corresponds with his character's trip down an elevator shaft after crossing the soap opera's writers. And the fleeting profound thought signifies his refusal to obsess over complex ideas and conflicted emotions. That, or it's a red herring.

The scheme: Roll with the punches. This may sound a lot like go with the flow, but there's a crucial difference. Unlike Phoebe, Joey possesses zero self-awareness. Think of it as the difference between a swimmer and a boxer. When swimmers go with the flow, they still have to know where they are in the water, concentrate on their breathing, and so on. Boxers operate on pure instinct. Between punches, they're doing what comes most naturally to us all—getting out of the way of a flying fist. Half the time, boxers aren't even conscious when they lose, so their egos sidestep a lot of bruising, too. Subsequently, Joey's wardrobe is an extension of his tough, indomitable sensibility. He flexes his muscles in masculine shades of black and olive; he works the Foosball machine in pugnacious pumpkin. Even the make of his clothing smacks of audacity—in real life, many of his garments far exceed his fictional means. For example, "The leather jacket Joey wore when he was unemployed was Armani," says McGuire. "Obviously, he couldn't have afforded it; I just wanted a leather jacket for him, and Armani had the best one. It wasn't supposed to read as 'Armani,' though, it was simply supposed to convey 'black leather.'" Got that? In fact, McGuire acknowledges that across the board, "I don't always dress the characters in clothes that necessarily suit their budgets, but I'm conscious as to how they're perceived visually. This is fantasy—that's the way it should be on TV. My main objective is to make the actors feel good, feel happy, and look great."

It's like a wonderful dream.

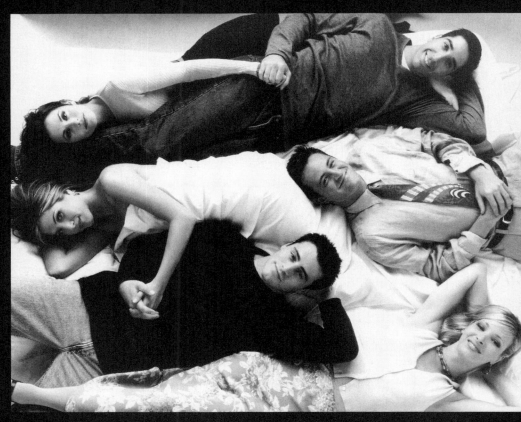

We're friends! And we're in bed together! 'Cause that's the kind of *Friends* we are! Starting with the fabulous body on top: Monica (Courteney Cox) does her very best to look casual and comfortable even though the bed's unmade; Ross (David Schwimmer) sports a schleppy Simian look (but will he do it for three more years?); Rachel (Jennifer Aniston) gets short-sheeted after her "accidental" naked photo shoot for *Rolling Stone*; Chandler (Matthew Perry) smiles like the cat who pressed his head up against the canary's butt; Joey (Matt LeBlanc) relaxes and thinks of bright shiny objects; and Phoebe (Lisa Kudrow) is the hippiest chick of all.

Quiz: Which Friend Are You?

Being a good friend means always being there for your pals, in rain, like before, etc. Being a good *Friend,* however, means pulling in the same big bucks as your fellow actors, getting an equal number of joke lines, and, oh yeah, wearing stylish outfits that highlight your individual, fabulously distinct personality. And while being a true friend is certainly important, knowing what kind of *Friend* you are is arguably even more crucial. Let's face it: Diet Coke doesn't give a rat's ass whether you send flowers to someone's sick aunt in the hospital or water your roommate's plants when she's on vacation. To get the big endorsements, you need to have network charisma. Luckily, inside all of us, there's a charismatic *Friend* screaming to get out. Which one? Take this quiz and see.

Part I: Are you a Monica, Rachel, or Phoebe?
1. You've got a big date tonight. This could be the night that the two of you finally do it—what do you wear?

    a) A cute little short-sleeved gray jersey A-line dress with black tights and heeled oxfords. A black handbag that holds your portable umbrella (in case it rains), an extra pair of tights (in case you get a snag), dental floss (in case you order spareribs), and a few tampons (in case). Also, fresh, clean white cotton panties—older guys dig that.

    b) Hard to say. On the chakra spectrum, the reds, greens, violets, and blues are feeling particularly strong. Which means . . . you'll wear them all!

    c) Short skirt, short shirt, and a shortcake short-cut for a short-term short stop with a tall, cool stranger. Whatever that means.

    d) A crocheted vest, some long gold chains, and a scarf around your head.

2. Another Sunday afternoon at Central Perk. You're not in the mood to fuss, so you figure you'll just hang out in:

a) Jeans and a short-sleeved turtleneck. Of course, you'll iron the jeans first.

b) A bright print top, and a long, flowing skirt. You can't distract the audience with too much leg when you're playing the guitar—they might not listen to the important words.

c) A geometric black-and-white stretch shirt, and a black miniskirt. Oh, and an apron. Or not.

d) Wide-legged pants, a patterned silk blouse, and knee-high zip-up boots. And a scarf around your head.

3. You're going for a job interview. You really want this job. After much deliberation, you finally decide on:

a) The most precious little red suit that has a fitted jacket with a bunch of adorable buttons down the front, and fourteen copies of your résumé.

b) Bell-bottoms, leggings, a dress—you know, what you'd normally wear. If they can't accept you for you, this wasn't meant to be.

c) A sleeveless dress with a matching jacket. It's the only thing that's clean right now. By the way, which job interview is this again?

d) A peasant-style floral dress, platform shoes, and a belted trench coat. And a scarf around your head. No, neck. No, head.

If you answered A to all of the above, you're a Monica. The good news is, with a body like that, you can wear anything. The bad news is, with all the time it takes to maintain a body like that, who has time to shop? Future projects: Figuring out how to get cast in another Jim Carrey movie, so you can buy a few more houses.

If your answers were all B, you're a Phoebe. Fortunately, your clothes are the most forgiving, body-wise; unfortunately, your clothes are the most demanding, style-wise. Future projects: Landing a major film role—right after you scrub off that damn milk mustache.

All you C-girls out there—are you ready to Rachel? Upside: You've got the look that everyone wanted to know better. Downside: And then they did. Future projects: Threatening to sue Rolling Stone *for putting that almost-naked photo of you on the cover that you "forgot" you posed for.*

And if you took the D-track, congratulations—you're a Rhoda. Luckily, it's better than being a Brenda. Unluckily, it's not as good as being a Mary. Future projects: Working your way up to three square meals a day.

Part II: Are you a Ross, Joey, or Chandler?

1. You've got a big date tonight. This could be the night that the two of you finally do it—what do you wear?

a) A retro Structure sweater that zips up the front over a T-shirt, and a pair of jeans. Not that it matters—the night'll probably be a total bust anyway.

b) Black jeans, a white T-shirt, and your lucky oversize tan-checked sport jacket—younger chicks dig that.

c) Khakis, a deep blue button-down shirt, and a natty sport coat. Sigh.

d) Starched white shirt, short white jacket, crisp white pants with a crease that could slice bread, and a white hat on your head.

2. Another Sunday afternoon at Central Perk. You're not in the mood to fuss, so you figure you'll just hang out in:

a) A T-shirt, sweatshirt, sweat jacket, sweatpants. Not that anyone cares.

b) An olive cotton Henley T-shirt and jeans. You got a problem with that?

c) Khakis, a dark green button-down shirt, and a nubbly tweed sport coat. Sigh.

d) Short-sleeved white shirt and crisp white pants with a crease that could spread butter. And a white hat on your head.

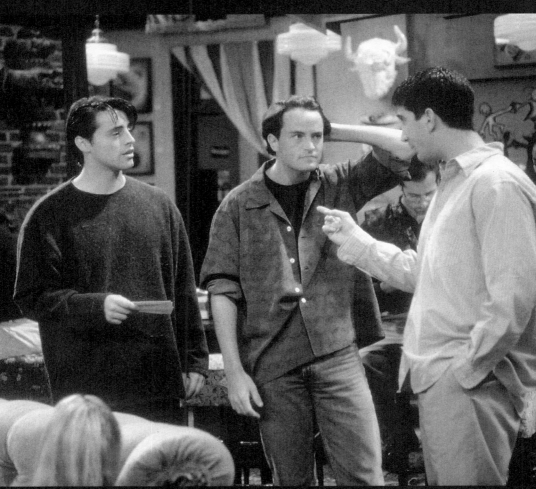

Three's the charm. The boy *Friends*, starting with that handsome lug on the left: Joey (Matt LeBlanc) wears his heart on his very, very long sleeves; Chandler (Matthew Perry) proves that he, his clothes and his hair are all multi-layered; and Ross (David Schwimmer) points out that he was once the highest-paid member of the cast. With friends like that, who needs *Seinfeld*?

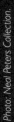

3. You're going for a job interview. You really want this job. After much deliberation, you finally decide to go with:

    a) A slate blue Hugo Boss suit, white shirt, and a conservatively radical print tie. Not that they'll hire you.

    b) Dark orange rayon shirt, black jeans, a black leather jacket, headshots, and a few extra condoms.

    c) Five-button Paul Smith taupe suit and bright green shirt. Heavy sigh.

    d) Blinding white shirt, white jacket with extra-special gold bars and buttons, and white pants with a crease that could carve a whole roasted pig. And a white hat on your head. No, under your arm. No, on your head.

If you got all A's, welcome to the Chandler zone of negativity—you'll get the job, but you won't get the girl. Future projects: You already dated Julia Roberts—what more do you want?

On the B-list, you're riding the Joey happy-go-dumb-lucky wave—you'll get the girl, but you won't get the job. Future projects: Ed II—This Time, It's Equine.

All you C-boys out there—are you ready to Ross? If so, you'll get the job and the girl and possibly a chronic case of hiccups from all that sighing.

And on the D-list, ahoy there, mateys—it's Captain Steubing! Forget the job, forget the girl, you've got a ship to steer! Future projects: Uh, not to nit-pick, but they're not just projects. They're the love *projects.*

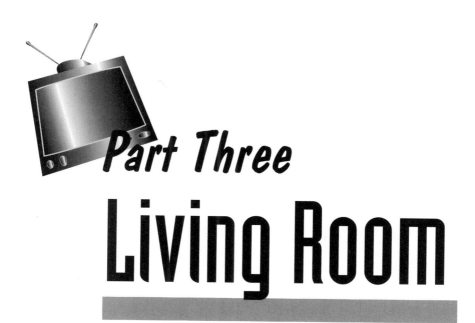

Part Three
Living Room

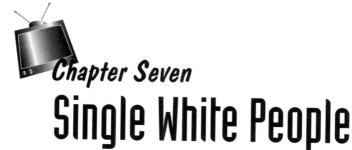

Chapter Seven
Single White People

Tuesday, 9:30 P.M. (NBC) CAROLINE IN THE CITY

(1995–present). Comely, young cartoonist from the Midwest moves to New York and fills the small screen with artsy Downtown togs. Motley crew of friends accompany her on her quest to meet that special someone. More perky than hip.

Monday, 9:30 P.M. (CBS) CYBILL

(1994–present). Plucky, aging actress tries to keep head above water in Los Angeles, and fills the small screen with medium-gloss California glamor. Two ex-husbands, two daughters, and one best friend accompany her on her quest to meet that special someone. More upbeat than clever.

Thursday, 8:30 P.M. (NBC) THE SINGLE GUY

(1995–present). Strapping novelist seeks literary fame in New York, and fills the small screen with tailored trends. Array of married friends and lovable doorman accompany him on his quest to meet that special someone. More hip and perky than upbeat and clever.

Wednesday, 8:00 P.M. (ABC) ELLEN

(1994–present). Bookstore employee-turned-owner cracks wise in Los Angeles, and fills the small screen with eclectic mod-squad style. Friends, family, and employees are accompanied by her on their quests to meet that special someone. More hip, perky, upbeat, and clever than any of the rest.

sn't it a drag when you go to dinner with a new guy, run into all your friends on the street and get mugged en masse? Or when your blind date turns out to be a Mafia princess and all your friends have to covertly follow you around town to make sure you don't get rubbed out? Or when you enlist a friend to rescue you from an anticipated fix-up from Hell, and then you end up really liking the guy and you can't get rid of your friend? What's that? Stuff like this never happens to you? Yeah, us neither. It does, however, happen to Caroline and Johnny and Cybill and Ellen. Because, you know, *they're on television.*

Yes, folks, it's a bright new day in Sitcom City, where the gang's all here and they aren't budging from your side, no sirreebob. You can't date with 'em, you can't date without 'em, you probably can't even go to the bathroom without 'em (which is why you never see anyone going to the bathroom on TV, because how are they supposed to fit you and the gang plus a whole camera crew in one little loo?). Even so, you love 'em, you need 'em, and you're nothing without 'em. Conclusion: If you want a hit, you've gotta have some major "'em." Why do you think they're called the Emmys? (Come to think of it, why are they called the Emmys?) On prime time, one-person shows just don't make the cut. *An Evening with Mark Twain?* Nielsen nightmare. *Medea?* Not even a summer replacement. *'Em Butterfly?* Huge.

Of course, you can't settle for just any old "'em." There has to be a certain look, a certain flair, a certain *nous ne savons quoi.* Actually, we do *savons quoi* (after several hundred hours of interviewing costume designers and watching TV, we damn well better *savons quoi*).

When you're searching for your own personal 'em, you want a group of people who don't overpower your fashion sense but can stand on their own. Who don't clash with your style but rather, complement it. Essentially, you'd look for "'em" the same way you'd look for, oh, say, that special someone. As such:

Desperately Seeking Laughs—"This Time, It's Personals."

Desperately Seeking Laughs personals service is a weekly feature. Cost is two minutes per punch line, half hour minimum. Approximately five to seven characters equal one show. Fashion references and sartorial background information must accompany ad order. Ad will run for twenty-six weeks; depending on response, may continue into syndication. Desperately Seeking Laughs is not responsible for any style errors or omissions. Limited abbreviations, please.

SWG [single, white guy/girl] seeks **BFF** [best female friend] to support inevitably doomed dating choices and subsequently provide comfort during inevitable doom-invoked gloom. Must like late-night partying, coffee, leather, high heels, fitted jackets, heavy drinking/smoking, and have experience in doling out free advice. Visual contrast with SWG a must.

List of Candidates:
Name: Annie (Amy Pietz).
Address: *Caroline in the City*.
Occupation: *Cats* dancer—the now-and-forever kind.
Preoccupation: Indiscriminate sex—the right-now and not-even-close-to-forever kind.
Character profile: Long Island working-class girl takes bite out of the Big Apple and spits it out clear across the Hudson.

Fashion profile: More trendy than sophisticated. Stretch corduroy jeans, hip-huggers, and bold print pants embrace Annie's lower half. Although she doesn't love dresses, she has been known to frock on a first date. As for her upper half, "Amy really does have a dancer's body," says *Caroline* costume designer Elizabeth Palmer, "so we put her in formfitted T-shirts, leotards, and stretch-velvet halters. She looks especially good in colors like burgundy, green, black, and brown, because her eyes and hair are dark—pale tones tend to wash her out." To complete the picture, she wears big, clunky jewelry (if any) and big, clunky shoes (again, if any).

Trademark: Black leather pants and jacket, not to mention her ubiquitous ratty blue terry-cloth bathrobe.

Likes: A good stiff drink, but only if it's after noon.

Dislikes: Getting out of bed anytime before noon.

Name: Maryann (Christine Baranski).

Address: *Cybill.*

Occupation: Lady who lunches.

Preoccupation: Primping, preening, polishing, and coiffing, so she can look *just so* at lunch. But first, a little shopping.

Character profile: Flip, flamboyant, and acidic as can be; if she were a litmus test, she'd stop traffic. All the gold plate in the world can't gild a pill like her—but underneath it all, she's a pretty good pill.

Fashion profile: More flash than substance. "Her character is slightly mad, and the clothes are pretty wild," says founding *Cybill* costume designer, Robert Turturice. "In fact, I think what she wears reflects the slight madness that exists in fashion today. You can't go too far with Maryann." For instance, she loves theme outfits: consider the Italian street-walker look—complete with black leggings, very high-heeled black strappy sandals, and a goldenrod sweater with

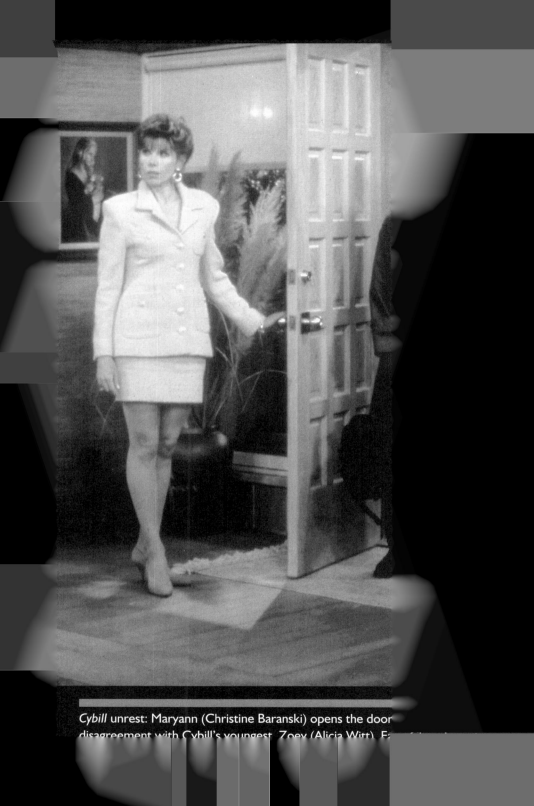

Cybill unrest: Maryann (Christine Baranski) opens the door
disagreement with Cybill's youngest, Zoey (Alicia Witt). F....

coq feathers lining the cuffs. Fabric-wise, it's a free-for-all: fuzzy leopard spots, animal-print trims, snakeskin, gabardine, and everything in between. "She's worn thigh-high boots with a formfitting body suit," says Turturice. "She'll put on the most outrageous runway fashion that you'd ordinarily look at and think, 'Who the hell would ever wear *that?*'"

Trademark: Designer brand names—for more! Nonetheless, although Maryann could conceivably afford to Chanel-surf, she has been known to *faux* on the first date. When she's feeling original, she leans primarily on Yves St.-Laurent, Stuart Weitzman, and Lagerfeld. "Lacroix colors work well on her," says Turturice, "especially bright yellow, hot pink, baby pink, red, orange." This is not a quiet woman.

Likes: A good stiff drink, but not before lunch.

Dislikes: Breakfast.

Name: Paige (Joely Fisher).

Address: *Ellen.*

Occupation: Rising Hollywood executive.

Preoccupation: The endless fascination that is Paige.

Character profile: Barbie meets Wild Irish Rose.

Fashion profile: More feminine than, uh, Ellen. To even out the *sui* DeGeneres menswear look, Paige is all girly-girl. "We make her look deliberately feminine, in contrast to Ellen," says Bambi Breakstone, costume designer for the show. "We start with tight, soft, sensuous fabrics and bright colors like green, cream, rust, turquoise. She usually wears a lot of angora, cashmere sweaters from Calvin Klein, and silk print dresses; when she's working, she's in short skirts and fitted jackets with open blouses." Even her casual look is ultra-fem: Cigarette pants from Bisou Bisou with a lacy blouse tucked in, silk shirts knotted at the waist, and mules or go-go boots.

Trademark: Hair so red it matches Maryann's litmus test.

Likes: A good stiff guy on parade.

Dislikes: Ellen's tendency to rain on that parade.

SWG seeks **BMF** [best male friend] to provide crucial insight into the male POV and/or furnish hilarious impressions of "what women think." Must dress almost exclusively in outdated clothing. Strange hair, wrinkled shirts, chinos, floppy sneakers and a know-it-all attitude are definite assets.

List of Candidates:

Name: Richard (Malcolm Gets).

Address: *Caroline in the City.*

Occupation: Struggling artist.

Preoccupation: Snuggling cartoonist.

Character profile: Deep, in an artsy, surface sort of way.

Fashion profile: More affected than effected. "This past season, our main concept for Richard was Starving Artist," says Palmer. "We kept him in all black, or varying shades of black." For contrast within the monochromatic scheme, Palmer used layers, textures, and subtle patterns—e.g., a nubby wool jacket over a retro-style striped shirt. Like *Seinfeld*'s Kramer, Richard gets most of his shirts either at vintage stores, or wears new reproductions of the same old, same old.

Trademark: Raincoat that ostensibly reflects his depressed, cynical, tortured soul. "It's long, dark and menacing," says Palmer. Along with those heavy tortoiseshell glasses, it manages to tone down the J. Crew–model effect quite nicely.

Likes: Caroline.

Dislikes: Liking Caroline.

Name: Sam and Trudy (Joey Slotnick and Ming-Na Wen).

Address: *The Single Guy.*

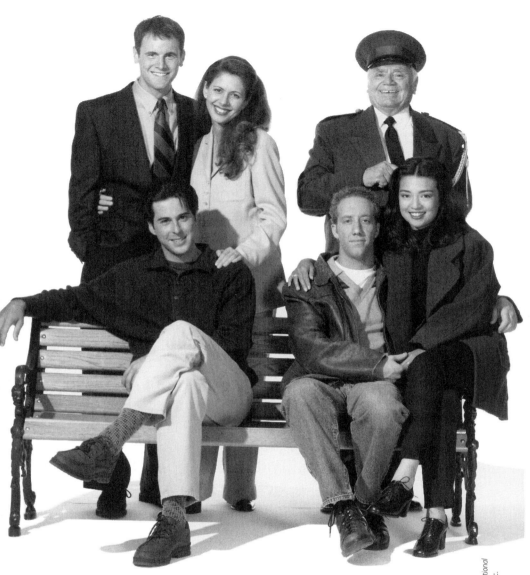

One! Singular sensation—every little cast change they make. *The Single Guy* circa 1995, clockwise from the sexy, smouldering uniformed man at top right: Manny (Ernest Borgnine) is forever Marty; Trudy (Ming-Na Wen) is the token Artisan; Sam (Joey Slotnick) is the token Music Mixer; Johnny (Jonathan Silverman) has a rocket in his pocket; and Matt and Janine (Mark Moses and Judith Hecht) are simply . . . dispensable.

Occupation: Sam's a record producer; Trudy has a mystery job in the art world (funny how she never ran into Richard, what with all that cross-over business going on last season).

Preoccupation: Convincing their Outer Nerds and Inner Cool People to swap places.

Character profile: Ho meets Hum (you can decide who's who). Oh, they try to carry off the illusion of having edge, but frankly, this kind of edge can't even spread the mustard, much less cut it.

Fashion profile: Sam went to college with Jonathan, and he doesn't seem to have bought many clothes in the interim. His "creative" career allows him to slouch on the casual side, in tennis shoes, khakis, rayon plaid shirts, baggy jackets, and a leather car coat. "He's happy in Ralph Lauren and Banana Republic," says Simmons, "because they carry retro styles, and have great blazers and sweaters." As a natural carrot-top, his color palette is limited; Simmons sticks with black or other dark neutrals—which ties in neatly with his rock-world affiliation. Although wife, Trudy, looks good in almost any color, she wears a lot of black, too (it's an art-world thing). She generally makes the scene in slip dresses, longer skirts, tight pants, sleeveless sweaters, and tops from designers like Nicole Miller and Donna Karan. Her boots or shoes always have a healthy heel, and her jewelry is eclectic, as though she could have picked it up in a Soho bazaar. Back when Soho *had* bazaars.

Trademark: His-and-hers leather coats—oooh, *edgy.*

Likes: Getting all dressed up to complain.

Dislikes: Getting any deeper than that.

Name: Spence (Jeremy Piven).

Address: *Ellen.*

Occupation: Almost a doctor, almost a lawyer, now very much a permanent houseguest.

Preoccupation: Freeloading.

Character profile: Moody, sarcastic, confused, with asocial tendencies. You know—everybody's ex-boyfriend.

Fashion profile: More less than more. The idea with Spence is that he arrived on Ellen's doorstep with one suitcase that held one basic shirt, one basic pair of pants and one sport coat. And while he's expanded since then, he's pretty much always wearing one of these key items. Once again, his style is vintage-redux: "Most of his shirts are from the fifties," says Breakstone. "I go to secondhand stores like American Rag as well as costume warehouses."

Trademark: Khakis in lieu of jeans—Spence has a half dozen of them from Kikit, in different earth tones. Six great pants, one nondescript look.

Likes: Poking merciless fun at people.

Dislikes: People.

SWG seeks **ESO** [ex–significant other] to remind her of previous relationship errors. Must be fluent in I-told-you-so-ese. Should have potential for brief sexual dalliance with SWG in moment of extreme weakness and vulnerability, but then be able to explain that said dalliance was merely another mistake to add to her collection. References requested.

List of Candidates:

Name: Del (Eric Lutes).

Address: *Caroline in the City.*

Occupation: Newspaper mogul—Caroline's ex-fiancé and current boss.

Preoccupation: His own dashing good looks.

Character profile: Egotist with a heart. You know, everybody's second husband.

Fashion profile: More pomp than circumstance. The essence of male vanity, Del favors double-breasted Armani and Canali suits. His color scheme is "the mud range," says Palmer. "We coordinate the suit and tie, and add a crisp white shirt for contrast—white looks great against his olive skin. He really is a gorgeous man." Yes, but can he act?

Trademark: Basic black . . . Porsche.

Likes: Caroline. On and off.

Dislikes: Richard. On and on.

Name: Grant (Tom Wopat) and Ira (Alan Rosenberg).

Address: *Cybill.*

Occupation: Grant is a Hollywood stunt man, Ira is a novelist. Same diff.

Preoccupation: Where their next job is coming from.

Character profile: Grant is a good-natured womanizer who lives by the seat of his pants. Ira is a good-natured nebbish who lives on the seat of his pants.

Fashion profile: A rotating collection of five flannel or denim work shirts, five pairs of jeans, and five pairs of sweat socks make up Grant's entire wardrobe—he may not quite live up to the "bubbly" feel of the show (as Turturice describes it), but he's in only about thirteen episodes a season. Ira is quietly resplendent in sweats, grungy shirts, pants, and jackets. "Ira's a human unmade bed," says Turturice. "He's a mess. He never matches and his clothes are utilitarian—he's always half pulled together in muted colors." Then again, Ira is a writer, and everyone knows that writers are the biggest slobs on earth (present company excluded—we're actually high-fashion models in our spare time, don't you know?).

Trademark: Grant: biceps; Ira: bicarbs.

Likes: Hanging out with each other, and former wife like one big, weird happy family.

Dislikes: Any implication that behavior such as this *might not be entirely normal.*

SWG seeks **WS** [wacky sidekick] to provide comic relief during half hour of . . . comedy? Whatever. Offbeat clothes, odd nasal patterns, and funny hats a plus. Humorous gimmick a requisite. Plotwise, should be prepared to take a backseat to the action. No babies or pets, please.

List of Candidates:

Name: Charlie (Andy Lauer).

Address: *Caroline in the City*.

Occupation: Errand boy for Del.

Preoccupation: Trying to get a plot line.

Fashion gimmick: More *porter* than *prêt*. You see, the guy's perpetually wearing sweatshirts and Rollerblades—at weddings, at funerals, in cars, at bars. Wherever he goes, he's rolling. Rolling up, rolling down. Rolling, rolling, rolling . . . RAWHIDE!

Name: Zoey (Alicia Witt).

Address: *Cybill.*

Occupation: Daughter/student.

Preoccupation: Trying to protest a plot line.

Fashion gimmick: More sourpuss than sex kitten. Zoey's a rebel without a tailor—she layers overdyed, oversized, unstructured garments in dark, saturated-color clothes to cocoon her from the crass commercialistic looks-obsessed world she hates. She's a television dream!

Name: Manny (Ernest Borgnine).

Address: *The Single Guy.*

Occupation: Guarding the fort.

Preoccupation: Trying to get through an entire plot line without any scary flashbacks to the *Poseidon Adventure*.

Fashion gimmick: More of the same. For some curious reason, his entire wardrobe consists of a gray six-button jacket, gray trousers with red piping, and a matching cap—hey, wait a minute, that's a doorman's uniform! Just who do you think you're trying to fool here?

Name: Joe (David Anthony Higgins) and Audrey (Clea Lewis).

Address: *Ellen.*

Occupation: Joe's the cappuccino man, Audrey's the stock girl, and they're both stock characters, we'll tell you that for free.

Preoccupation: Trying to trip up the plot line.

Fashion gimmick: For Joe, more poi than polloi. Hawaiian shirts are his funny, funny uniform, along with great big jeans. He will wear them on a train, he will wear them in the rain. In a house, with a mouse, in a box, with a fox—why, he would wear them in a tree, they are so bright, so *right,* you see! For Audrey, more pink than anything else. She lives *la vie en rose* (with a little *blanc* thrown in); the sixties silhouette includes Mary Quant-esque baby-doll dresses, mohair sweaters, pedal pushers, miniskirts and hair bows. Giving her the blush-off consumes a lot of Breakstone's time; what she can't find, she has to dye. "On one episode," recalls Breakstone, "Carol Kane played Audrey's mother. I thought it would be funny to have her dress all in lavender—you know, the color swatch doesn't fall far from the spool." GAP, Rampage, and Benetton are fertile shopping grounds, as are children's sections of department stores—Lewis is a size two-minus and can wear junior sizes easily. That little pink bitch.

SWG seeks self—otherwise, none of the above characters will have anything to do. Must be distinctive, likable, nonthreatening and, most of all, easy to relate to. No ultra-hip, strange, haute, or trendy fashion allowed—too intimidating. Self-deprecating humor a requirement. If first name can be used for sitcom title, all the better.

List of Candidates:

Name: Caroline Duffy (Lea Thompson).

Address: Well, that would be the City.

Occupation: Cartoonist.

Preoccupation: Meeting that special, special someone.

Character profile: So cute. So sweet. So kind. So lucky she got such a choice time slot that her cute, sweet, kind candy-ass didn't get plowed off the air.

Fashion profile: More over than powering. Caroline's no fashion maverick—she's a follower, not a leader. "We avoid big color and style statements," says Palmer. "Lea's features are so delicate and her coloring's so light, we have to be careful the clothes don't overwhelm her." Pastels work best: pale yellow, lavender, blue, teal, and sometimes richer burgundies and greens, but "white and off-white drain any rose out of her cheeks." To emphasize Caroline's girlish quality, Palmer will have her wear jeans with a shirt half-tucked in. You can, however, expect her to look more tailored as time goes by: the simpler, the better. "Flowery stuff on Caroline is out," says Palmer. "You'll see lots of T-shirts with jeans and blazers, and blouses with nice slacks from Jil Sander in Caroline's future. I'd like to get less body conscious and more classic." Long chains and antique jewelry pieces complete the romantic-novel approach. As for height, Thompson's diminutive size-four body gets a boost with chunky heeled shoe-boots.

Trademark: The schoolgirl headband, for two reasons. It keeps the hair out of her face, and "it's cute."

Likes: Being serious and cute, concerned and cute, distraught and cute, silly and cute.

Dislikes: Who cares about *her* dislikes? *We hate cute.*

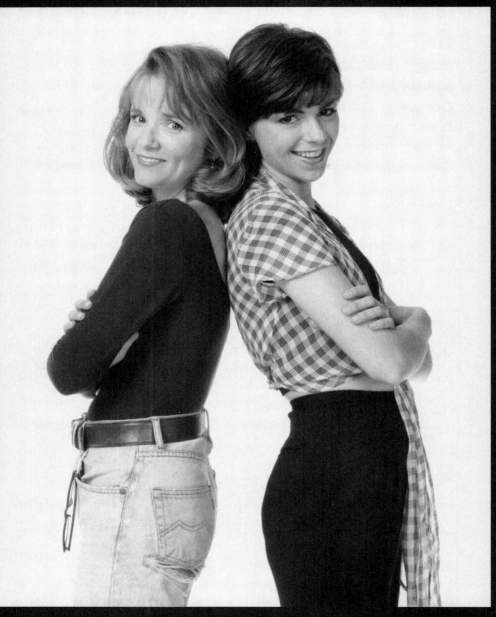

But how cute will they be when they're not back-to-back with *Seinfeld* and *ER*? Caroline (Lea Thompson) and Annie (Amy Pietz) put on their City duds, cross their arms and smile. And pray.

Name: Cybill Sheridan (Cybill Shepherd).

Address: Los Angeles, California.

Occupation: Actress and mother.

Preoccupation: Flushing out that special someone.

Character profile: Still going . . . 'cause she's not getting older, she's getting better!

Fashion profile: More grace than fire. "When we started out, the idea was eclectic and fun," says Turturice. "Knit vests with jeans, sweaters with high heels, Hawaiian shirts with leggings. When she goes out to lunch with Maryann, she opts for dressier separates, like pleated trousers with a fitted jacket. Sometimes her jackets are cropped, but we also did a riding jacket length on Cybill that looked great." Then again, in Turturice's eyes, it's all great. He adores buying fabulous designer duds (such as Escada, Emanuel, Bebe), then combining them with bargain-basement stuff. He has a ball mixing black with brights. "I love to put black jeans with a red jewel-tone top. I love jewel blues and green," he enthuses. "The whole show is sparkly and madly bright, so I picked clothes to go with that spirit." This is a man who enjoys his job. America salutes him.

Trademark: Animal slippers (namely fuzzy ducks, flamingos, alligators, and koalas). And pins. "Cybill always wears a little pin that looks artsy and handmade," comments Turturice. "Some are elaborate enamel things, but others are tiny little antique board-game pieces." Cute, but they ain't no headband.

Likes: Getting better.

Dislikes: Getting older.

Name: Johnny Elliot (Jonathan Silverman), a.k.a. The Single Guy.

Address: New York, New York.

Occupation: Wildly gesticulating novelist.

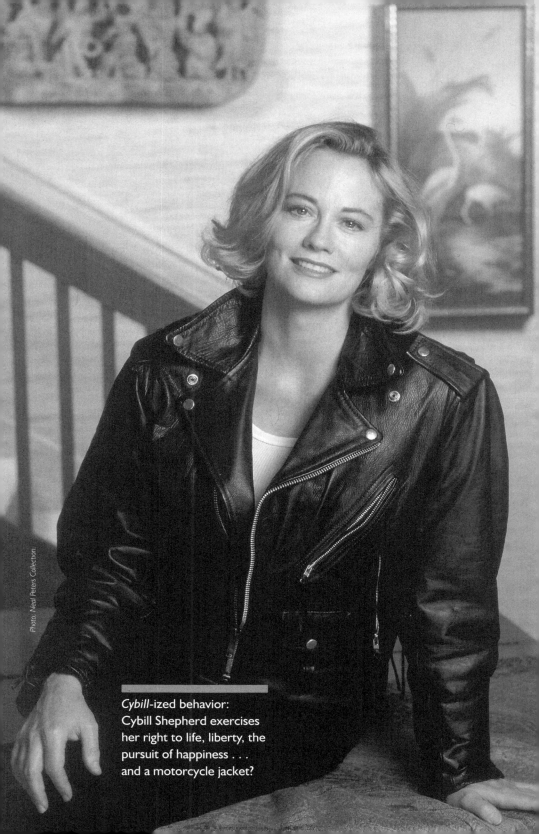

Cybill-ized behavior:
Cybill Shepherd exercises
her right to life, liberty, the
pursuit of happiness . . .
and a motorcycle jacket?

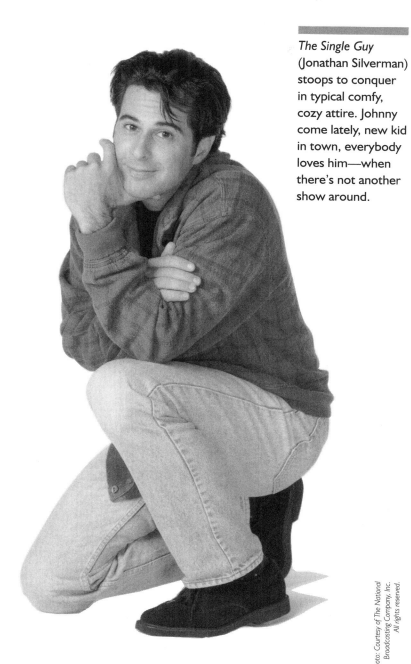

The Single Guy
(Jonathan Silverman)
stoops to conquer
in typical comfy,
cozy attire. Johnny
come lately, new kid
in town, everybody
loves him—when
there's not another
show around.

Preoccupation: Scaring off that special someone.

Character profile: Very *Biloxi Blues*, very *Weekend at Bernie's*, very . . . Jonathan Silverman. No matter how hard he tries, he just can't shake it.

Fashion profile: More that-was-then than this-is-now. Stylistically, this single guy hasn't changed much since his junior year of college, and for good reason. "He's supposed to be holding on to his bachelorhood," says Simmons, "so we put him in that kind of clothing." This means Lucky jeans with a little wider leg in less predictable colors (darker indigo, khaki, stone, brown), T-shirts under flannel long-sleeved shirts, and Reeboks. For dress-up occasions, he sharpens up with Armani blazers and slacks. "Except for the suits," says Simmons, "we want everything to look used or beat up—nothing in Jonathan's closet should look too new." It doesn't.

Trademark: Terminally tousled hair. Chicks dig it . . . don't they?

Likes: Having loved and lost.

Dislikes: Ever having loved at all.

Name: Ellen Morgan (Ellen DeGeneres).

Address: Los Angeles.

Occupation: Bookstore owner.

Preoccupation: Wondering why everyone around her is so obsessed with meeting that special someone. Special someone? What the hell is that supposed to mean?

Character profile: Friendly and dry as an unexpected martini at the end of a long day.

Fashion profile: More sense than sensibility. Other than the two minutes when she tried on a bridesmaid dress, Ellen stands resolutely in pants—mostly J. Crew or Banana Republic flat-front khakis (with the pockets sewn shut to keep them looking neat). When she puts on jeans, they're beat up Levi's 501s from used clothing stores. "We try to keep it simple,"

Be an *Ellen* degenerate—or just look like one.

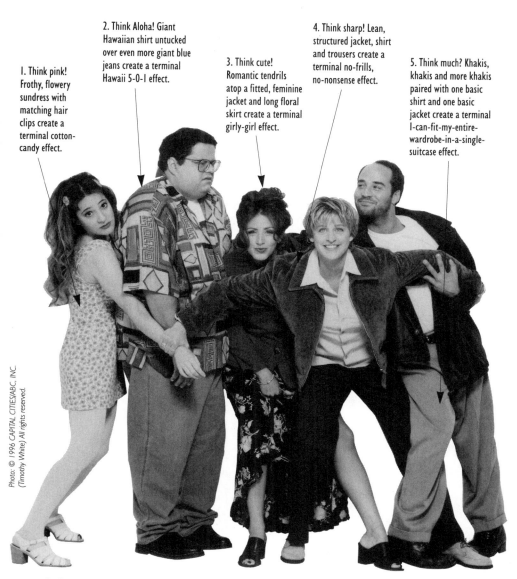

1. Think pink! Frothy, flowery sundress with matching hair clips create a terminal cotton-candy effect.

2. Think Aloha! Giant Hawaiian shirt untucked over even more giant blue jeans create a terminal Hawaii 5-0-1 effect.

3. Think cute! Romantic tendrils atop a fitted, feminine jacket and long floral skirt create a terminal girly-girl effect.

4. Think sharp! Lean, structured jacket, shirt and trousers create a terminal no-frills, no-nonsense effect.

5. Think much? Khakis, khakis and more khakis paired with one basic shirt and one basic jacket create a terminal I-can-fit-my-entire-wardrobe-in-a-single-suitcase effect.

Left to right: Audrey (Clea Lewis), Joe (David Anthony Higgins), Paige (Joely Fisher), Ellen (Ellen DeGeneres), Spence (Jeremy Piven) explains Breakstone. "We want an unadorned, untailored look that's still hip. Ellen wears T-shirts under lean, structured jackets and zip-up cardigans; she doesn't bother with frills or patterns besides pinstripes. She's a no-nonsense person." Her colors are equally no-nonsense: blues (which also bring out her lovely blue eyes), corals, beiges, tans, black, grays, and greens. In terms of baubles, Ellen does like silver jewelry, in the form of a bead necklace, tiny, demure earrings, and a cluster of several rings. And she wraps it all up with a brown Maxfield Parish double-breasted leather jacket.

Trademark: Originally famous for her all-occasion Adidas sneakers, last season, Ellen exclusively wore Hush Puppies in every color (white, powder blue, black, brown, and purple, to name a few). This year, she's stepping out in Vans. Optional title suggestion for the show: *These Trends of Mine.*

Likes: Subtle observational humor.

Dislikes: Unsubtle observational humor about her not being married. Everyone knows that marriage leads to kids, which leads to families, which—golly, who'da thunk—leads to **Chapter 8: Family Affairs**. (Okay, so it wasn't the most graceful transition on earth, but what do you want? It's almost Chapter 8—*we're tired.*)

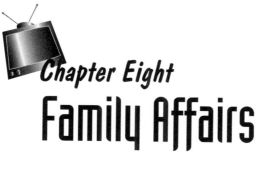

Chapter Eight
Family Affairs

SATURDAY, 9:00 P.M. (FOX) MARRIED . . . WITH CHILDREN

(1987–present). Story of a man named Bundy who is bringing up two very surly kids (along with wife, Peg). Lower-class slice of Chicago life; J.C. Penney–style comedy of bimbos and bargain-basement humor.

TUESDAY, 8:00 P.M. (ABC) ROSEANNE

(1988–present). Story of a broad named Roseanne who is bringing up three kids on her own (husband, Dan, recently jumped ship). Lower-middle-class slice of Illinois life; Sears-style comedy of muumuus and Milk Duds.

TUESDAY, 9:00 P.M. (ABC) HOME IMPROVEMENT

(1991–present). Story of a pair named Taylor, who are building up three tousle-headed boys. Middle-class slice of Detroit life; L.L. Bean–style comedy of hearth-and-home renovations.

WEDNESDAY, 8:00 P.M. (CBS) THE NANNY

(1994–present). Story of a lovely nanny, who is bringing up three kids, not her own (widowed father is too charmingly ineffectual to help). Upper-class slice of Manhattan life; Todd Oldham–style comedy of manicures and mayhem.

WEDNESDAY, 9:00 P.M. (ABC) GRACE UNDER FIRE

(1993–present). Story of a detoxed lady, who is stringing up three rough-and-ready kids (ex-husband, a wife-beating drunk, only appears in five episodes a season). Lower-middle-class slice of Missouri life. Salvation Army–style comedy of paying the bills and praying for sex.

WEDNESDAY, 9:00 P.M. (FOX) PARTY OF FIVE

(1994–present). Story of a brood named Salinger who is bringing up itself on its own (parents were killed by a drunk driver). Unclassified slice of San Francisco life; singular-style drama of coming to terms and coming of age.

Remember the old days, when the Bradys were your average on-screen family? And how domestic upheaval could be triggered by, say, Peter being cast as Benedict Arnold in a school play and no one speaking to him because it wasn't patriotic? Or by Cindy reading Marcia's diary? (Remember when people actually used the word *patriotic* and kept diaries?) Yeah, those were the days. Then, in real life, it turned out that Dad Brady probably had way more than three boys "of his own," that Greg was shanking his sisters off camera, and—poof!—the myth of the TV-perfect family disintegrated into more dust than Alice could shake a mop at.

Enter the New TV Family, in which sex, drugs, and rock and roll are status quo (the *quo* being optional) and where the problems are neither dressed up nor wrapped up within a half hour. What would Mike and Carol have said about Darlene's teen maternity clothes? Or Julia's miscarriage outfit on *Party of Five?* Or the myriad lovers Kelly Bundy has notched in her leather belt? Probably something along the lines of, "Good heavens!" A more accurate appraisal: good ratings.

And as the television family-values system shifts, so shifteth the fashions. Whether they're two-parent, one-parent, or no-parent homes, each situation has its own unique set of problems, its own unique look. No more of that "youngest one in curls" crap—in this modern age, both parents and kids have more signature style-statements than Cindy could shake a hairbrush at. Below, a roundup of moms, dads, surrogates, and kids—who they are and what they wear. And 'til the one day when Dan Quayle rules the airwaves, we know that it's much more than a hunch, that this group will redefine the family, in a way that's nothing like the BRADY BUNCH—THE BRADY BUNCH, THE BRADY BUNCH, THAT'S THE . . . anyway. You know the rest.

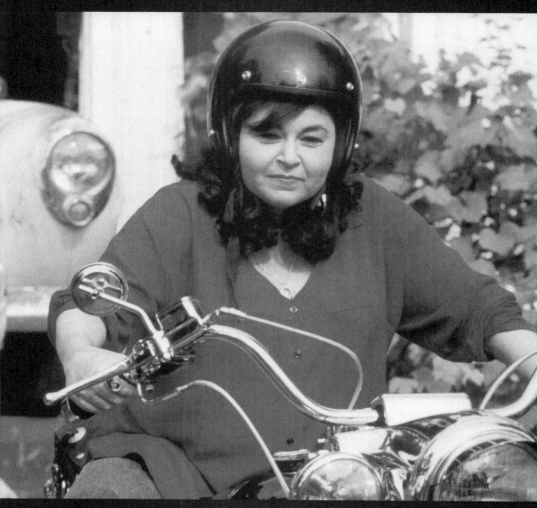

She-devil or Hell's Angel? Roseanne, the most famous mom in America, is all revved up for one more season on the motor(mouth)-cade.

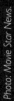

THE MOTHERS

All told, TV mothers both give and take the most. In front of the camera, they give advice, help, elbow grease, blood, sweat, tears, solace, shelter, and, uh, birth. Behind the scenes, though, they generally require the most time, effort, agony, and extra attention. Cool. Art really does imitate life.

Serial Mom: Roseanne Connor (Roseanne, the artist formerly known as Roseanne Arnold, formerly known as Roseanne Barr)/*Roseanne.* In the history of serial television moms, Roseanne has probably changed her look more times than anyone else—even more than the actress herself has changed her name. "Over the eight years we've been on the air, Roseanne's gone through a lot of styles," says costume designer Erin Quigley, "but we've always tried to maintain the spirit of her character." Clothing-wise, this translates to jewel tones which flatter her complexion, and styles with "vivacity" that fit her larger-than-life personality. First came the jeans-and-man's-shirt phase, which morphed into leggings and smocks. When she lost weight, she turned to more fitted trousers and floral dresses; during her pregnancy, she wore bright, baby-dollish frocks (um, make that dresses—this is not a woman who wears *frocks*). There was even a brief tailored period, although frankly it doesn't stand tall in our memories. As for working duds, she's served time in a polyester waitress uniform, a floor-sweeper-in-a-hair-salon jacket, a factory-shop jumper, and, of course, her apron at The Lunch Box. This season, now that she's got her own morning show, she'll pack her punches in spiffier jacket-and-skirt ensembles; she won't necessarily be more upscale, but definitely more pulled together. And while heels rarely make the scene, she has sneakers, slip-on flats, and Doc Martens galore.

So where do you shop for a 360-degree-turn woman? Anywhere you want. "I go everywhere, from mainstream chains like Nordstrom, Bullock's, and Neiman Marcus to tiny thrift stores and midwestern Sears," says Quigley. "When I want tacky and tasteless, I usually head for half-sized or maternity stores. For Darlene's wedding, I went to a shop called Fat City." Meanwhile, *Fat City?* What happened to politely euphemistic names like Charisma! or The Forgotten Woman? What's next—Lard Bodies? Crisco Kids? Come In And Buy Stuff Here, You Massive Load of Excess Flesh? Really.

One last note: Contrary to what those horrible media people report (and, boy, do we hate those horrible media people), "Roseanne is very easy to work with," says Quigley. "She doesn't care if she looks ugly, as long as it's right for the scene. This, to me, is the sign of a good actor." Sorry, Delta.

Cereal Mom: Peg Bundy (Katey Sagal) / *Married With . . . Children*. Let's be clear: Peg is not a woman who cooks. For starters, she'd ruin her nails. Plus, it would cut into her precious blow-drying hours. Besides which, she couldn't possibly cook in Those Shoes (you know, her ever-present mules with a Lucite high-heel, courtesy of Frederick's of Hollywood). One slip on a stray garlic clove, and she'd be history. And don't even begin to suggest that she go barefoot. She's been wearing them since the first episode! They're The Shoes that created The Walk! Have you no sense of history?

Nonetheless, however lacking in culinary skills, Peg is a veritable feast for the eyes. Not a fan of subtle neutrals, she pops in bright lime green, wild animal patterns like pink-and-black zebra, and on somber days, a basic leopard print. No square Peg, she. Up top, says costumer Marti Squires, the Peg-classic is a polyester, formfitting, low-cut long-sleeved shirt (Calypso ruffles and off-the-shoulder necklines optional), accented by a wide, waist-cinching belt. Down below, the Peg trademark is a pair of skintight Capri pants. Initially, they were polyester pull-ons with elastic waistbands from J.C. Penney. "I bought them in every color," says Squires. "With some hemming and a little flare added to the leg, I made them into the cropped pants she wears today." These days, Squires commissions the pants from the Bob Mackie Workshop. "We went from $19 at Penney's to $225 at Mackie's," observes Squires. "That's television." That's also entertainment. Throw in a fistful of gaudy necklaces, garish rhinestone earrings, and ridiculous shoe clips, and you've got a cornucopia of colors and textures that would take the edge off even the most peckish viewer's appetite. In this case, less is out of the question.

Stereo Mom: Jill Taylor (Patricia Richardson)/*Home Improvement*. Stereo-typical, that is. Jill Taylor is the most traditional mom of the group. Comfort is the operative word, usually in the shape of Levi's 501 jeans, flat-front, tapered trousers, crew-neck T-shirts, blouses, and tailored blazers. In the winter, she'll wear short skirts and tights, with a rust suede hip-length coat. And all year 'round, she's easy on the eye in jewel tones, neutrals, and brown (to match her pretty, shiny hair). Costume supervisor Nicole Gorsuch sticks mainly to vintage venues when she shops for Jill's jackets. "I look for items with details that can't be found in other stores," Gorsuch says. "Patricia looks good in a 1940s cut—it's an effective style for many women, because it draws attention to the shoulders, away from the hips." On her feet, she's never without a touch of heel. "Whether they're loafers or boots, they all have at least two-inch heels," says Gorsuch. "They make her long legs appear even longer." Her jewelry, too, is sweet and familiar—small pearl earrings or light stones

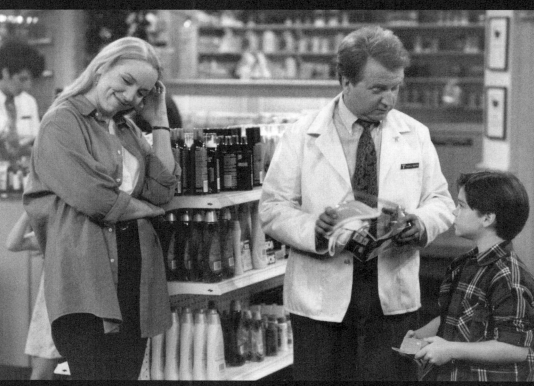

Grace Under Fire's Brett Butler (left) stands loosely by while Russell (Dave Thomas) explains the fine art of jock straps to Grace's son, Quentin (John Paul Steuer, right). That's what we call a family support system.

inside gold or silver settings. Mind you, despite the abundance of traditional garb, you'll never see this mommy in an apron, notonyourlifey. Even so, there's something about her that makes us feel all warm inside. Cozy. Snuggly. *Homey.*

Seminal Mom: Grace Kelly (Brett Butler) / *Grace Under Fire.* Sure, she may work in an oil refinery, but Grace also likes to consider herself a bit of an *artiste.* She paints. She writes. She attends poetry readings. And her clothes reflect her deep, deep nature. Over jeans, she'll wear hippie-chick, vintage-like unstructured shirts in rayon or crushed velvet—blue or black work best with her blond hair. She busts balls in overalls (coveralls at work), as well as oversized sweaters with leggings, and an infrequent floral dress. She hits the ground running in heeled work boots or DKNY loafers, and she ornaments herself with small, delicate antique earrings or hoops. Yup. She's a looker, all right. In fact she's hot, she's red hot, she's boiling hot, SHE'S UNDER FIRE! SHE'S UNDER FIRE! SHE'S UNDER—sorry. We don't know what came over us. It won't happen again.

Surreal Mom: Sylvia Fine (Renée Taylor) / *The Nanny.* As Fran's meshuga mother, Sylvia Fine is . . . a little hard to get over. Visualize a determined blond wig atop a size-sixteen body precariously perched on a tiny pair of high-heeled mules, and you pretty much get the picture. "She's got a big personality," says Brenda Cooper, costume supervisor for the show, "and she looks great in formfitted suits and big jewelry." That's some form to fit. Incidentally, whenever Fran and her mom are sharing the screen, they're a perfect color match. "I don't have a specific formula," Cooper says, "I just think of the palette and it comes together beautifully." An important element in dressing this over-the-top show, she adds, is a sense of humor. "The clothes should be funny in a witty way," declares Cooper. "Straight fashion on TV just looks stupid." Yeah, we know what she means. Especially on a *really intellectual show like The Nanny.*

THE FATHERS

Our quartet of fathers may get short sartorial shrift, but it goes a long way. From the upper crust to the bottom rung, these *paterfamilias* (that's Latin for "the old man") have serious visual impact (or should we say, *visualitas impactus?*). And that's all they need. Because on television, being a dad is more about serving as a figurehead, being a role model, and sustaining an image—without being burdened down by niggling day-to-day details. Art. Imitates. Life.

Deadbeat Dad: Al Bundy (Ed O'Neill) / *Married . . . With Children.* In fatherhood and clothinghood, Al Bundy occupies a class by himself—usually in plain brown shoes. "He's a very mundane character, so I keep him in a standard outfit: blue chambray dress shirt and brown polyester pants," says Squires. The shirts are such signature pieces that many fans have even asked him to autograph them. Yes, but can he write?

Deadwood Dad: Tim Taylor (Tim Allen) / *Home Improvement.* Unlike most of his counterparts, Tim actually has two different images: His Tool-Time look and his Not-Tool-Time look. The former, according to costume supervisor Valerie Laven-Cooper, is "peacocky, bold, and masculine." This means monochromatic outfits comprised of dark chambray shirts, Calvin Klein patterned ties, and pleated, cuffed slacks. The sport jackets he hands to Al are either matte or textured, from designers such as Zanella, Armani, Vestimenta, and Mel Fox. As for Not-Tool-Time Tim (say *that* ten times fast), why, he looks like every other fella in Detroit. "I want viewers to look at him and think, I'd like to wear that, too," says Laven-Cooper. If they did, it wouldn't be difficult to arrange: the lion's share of Tim's closet comes from catalogs and nationwide chains. Watch for J. Crew wide-wale corduroys, GAP easy-fit jeans and chinos, Banana Republic brown leather belts, L.L. Bean duck boots, and Eddie Bauer down vests. His footwear is strictly Nike. When he does venture a tad higher on the fashion food chain, you might see him in an Aviatrix brown bomber jacket or a Hugo Boss cotton windbreaker with a green-and-blue collar. Heartwarming sidebar: To support higher education in the state, Tim welcomes sweatshirts from all Michigan colleges. He contacts the schools, they send the sweatshirt, he wears it on the air, signs it, and sends it back for their promotional purposes. Uncle Tim wants U.!

Dead-calm Dad: Maxwell Sheffield (Charles Shaughnessy) / *The Nanny*. Playing the role of widowed dapper dad to the hilt, Maxwell Sheffield charms and delights in classic, contemporary styles. "I envision him trying to impress Fran by being hipper looking," says Cooper. "He's a well-dressed, dignified man of the arts." Plus, he's British, which makes him Mr. *Extra*-Fancy. Ergo, he sports three-piece suits (often in navy) by high-end designers such as Armani, Canali, and Donna Karan. "I like him in double-breasted," says Cooper. "When he's casual, he'll wear a suede jacket with monochromatic tones underneath. He's elegant, but never outlandish." When you're that rich, you can pay someone to be outlandish for you.

Dead Dad: Dan Connor (John Goodman) / *Roseanne*. Okay, he's not entirely dead (although he did have a heart attack at the end of last season), but he is only coming back part-time. Still, our full-time memories of him are warm, indeed. Toasty, in fact, since his wardrobe consists primarily of jeans and plaid flannel shirts. "We must have about two hundred

She's got a hairstyle *this big*. *The Nanny*'s Fran
(Fran Drescher) and Maxwell (Charles
Shaughnessy) are a stylish au pair, indeed.

plaid flannel shirts," says Quigley. Gosh, it must have been hell for him to pack and unpack. Work boots, Nikes, and Top-Siders clutter his closet floor; "He's worn the same pair of Top-Siders for seven or eight years," says Quigley. "I tried to convince him to wear a new pair, but he liked the old ones." Gift tip for next Father's Day? Odor Eaters.

THE SURROGATES

On the domesticated tube, a measly one or two parents isn't nearly enough. Hence, the networks provide families with surrogate parents (neighbors, relatives, hired help), who lend valuable child-rearing input—and offer a few proxy laughs in the process. Many hands make lite work. In this case, art takes such a drastic swing out of the realm of life, we're struggling to relate.

Tinkers: Al (Richard Karn) and Wilson (Earl Hindman)/*Home Improvement*. Tim's "Tool Time" partner and friend, Al is like an uncle to the kids. He's like a lumberjack to the viewers, in timeless red, green, and blue plaid flannel shirts (J. Crew and L.L. Bean), cuffed-at-the-bottom blue jeans (Banana Republic), and Red Wing boots. Off duty, he sticks with the plaid, but loses the flannel, with cotton or broadcloth shirts by Ralph Lauren and chinos. The scheme never varies, except when he goes on dates—at which point, he throws on a sweater. Help. We're swooning. Next-door neighbor Wilson is like a father figure to Tim, helping him whittle down life's quandaries with fortune-cookie wisdom and ten-cent nuggets of philosophy. He wears hats, therefore he is (you never see his face)—mostly fishing hats from L.L. Bean. Because he's usually outdoors, corduroy, wool, and down are favored materials. And because he's supposed to

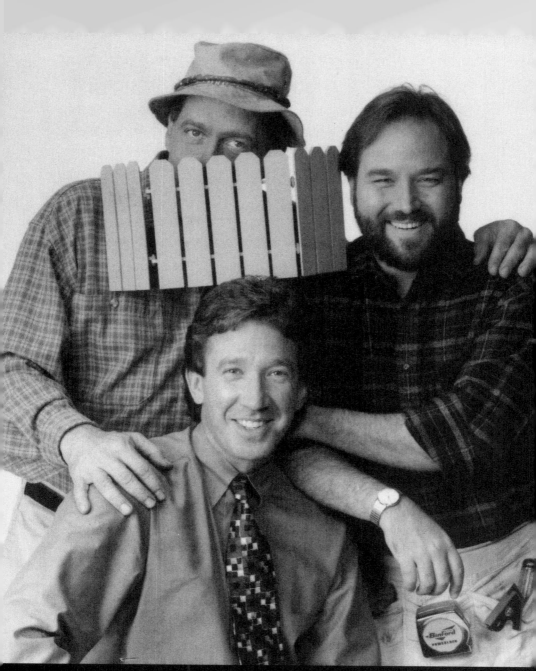

Meanwhile, back at the wrench. . . . *Home Improvement*'s trio of Real Men, starting from the guy with the picket fence hanging off his face: Wilson (Earl Hindman) checks in but keeps a low profile; Al (Richard Karn) measures up as Tim's "Tool Time" partner; and Tim (Tim Allen) ties the whole cast together.

be the wise and weathered sage, distressed chinos and earth tones are priorities. Ancient TV secret.

Tailored: Fran Fine (Fran Drescher)/*The Nanny*. In the Sheffield home, Fran is like a mother to the kids. Interestingly, this is the one show where the proxy parent also happens to be the star—and, honey, we're talking star with a capital S-T-A-W. This nanny would never hang out with a professor (too humdrum, too underpaid); she's intent on erasing the S from hometown Queens and making it her full-time occupation. In the meantime, she sits—and struts—for Maxwell Sheffield's trio of unbearably precious tots. "My departure point is glamour—Rita Hayworth, Katharine Hepburn— total glamour," says Cooper. "Whether the character's playing golf or doing business [commonplace nanny pursuits, mind you], the outfit should be polished from head to toe. I love Todd Oldham; he marches to the beat of the same drummer I march to." So much so that Oldham sporadically appears on the show as Fran's cousin, Toddy, who's—what else?—a garmento. Other designers in the cavalcade include Dolce & Gabbana, Moschino, and Isaac Mizrahi. Cooper also scans the department stores for one-of-a-kind outfits, like a rubber dress and matching coat from Loehmann's.

Of course, there's more to Nannyfication than merely throwing a couture schmatte over Fran's size-four shoulders. "I have to cobble together and coordinate the complete outfit," says Cooper. "That's where my art comes in." (Hey, don't look at us that way; we just report this stuff.) "Art" entails monitoring every stitch, from the tippy-top of Fran's imposing coif to the base coat of her pedicure. Along the way, you're usually treated to a major thoroughfare of leg. To streamline the trip, Cooper tailors every garment. "If I buy something that isn't fitted, I tailor it to fit. There's not

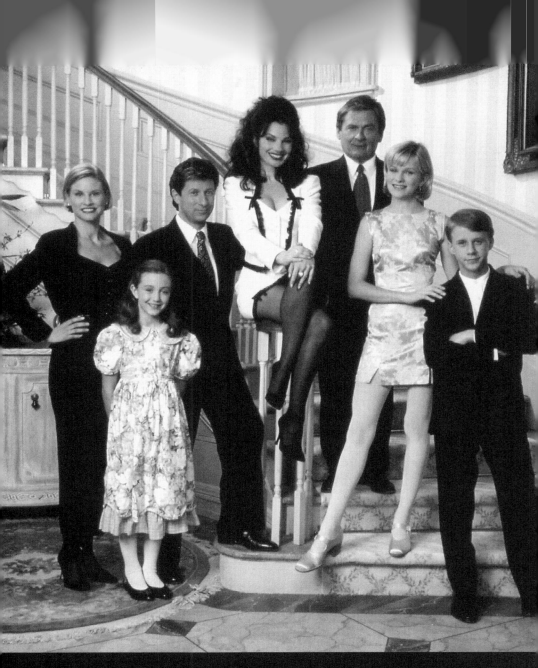

A photo awp with *The Nanny* pack. The Sheffield brood demonstrates their version of a twelve-step program, with Fran (Fran Drescher, sitting center) riding the designer rail, while father Maxwell (Charles Shaughnessy) stands one piece on the show that hasn't been altered." On the color spectrum, Fran can leap from hot pink to tartan in a single episode. "As long as it's sassy and sexy," Cooper declares, "it works." Hats are *verboten* and jewelry is minimal (except for Drescher's own stacked rings, which she sometimes forgets to remove), but bright red lipstick is a constant. And underneath it all, Drescher hides a—gasp—padded bra. "It makes the clothes fall better," says Cooper. "She never leaves home without it." Mental note for future: Surprise Fran at home.

Soldier. Jackie (Laurie Metcalf) / *Roseanne.* Roseanne's long-embattled kid sister, Jackie, is like an aunt to the kids. Come to think of it, she *is* an aunt to the kids. Like her older, bigger sibling, she, too, has experienced a series of clothing evolutions. Guess it runs in the family. "She started out dressing seductively," says Quigley, "in a cheap, midwestern, bad-hair kind of way. Now, as a new mother, she's more casual in jeans and Eddie Bauer oversized sweaters." A few of those sweaters are conversation pieces unto themselves—for example, the aqua Michael Simon number that bore the image of a bunch of Rastafarians in a bus ("We got a million calls about that one," remembers Quigley). Metcalf has a taste for the southwestern (Mexican swing coats, Native American patterns, etc.); "She can wear ethnic clothes," Quigley says. "She's more experimental than Roseanne." Like Roseanne, however, she looks best in vivid colors. Guess it runs in the—hey, hold on one little minute. They're not really related! We were born at night, but not last night!

Pry. Marcie D'Arcy (Amanda Bearse) / *Married . . . with Children.* Wife of Jefferson, neighbor of Al and Peg, Marcie is like an annoying cousin from another planet to the kids. That would be the Planet Someone's-gotta-dress-like-a-normal-person-on-this-show, natch. Since she works at a bank, she tends toward corporate-looking suits; even at home, she's well turned out, in pleated pants, blouses, and vests. "She's the one character I spend money on," says Squires. "Her suits are Armani, Donna Karan, and Anne Klein." So wait, what about Peg's Capri pants that cost $225 a shot? Heh? Betcha thought we weren't paying attention, didn't you?

THE KIDS

No Marcias or Gregs in this crowd: these kids are too intent on rebelling, recovering, and revamping to be bothered with any Rebecca of Sunnybrook Farming. And it shows in their clothes. Rugged individualists to the marrow, they march to the beat of a drummer that Todd Oldham hasn't even heard of yet (and when he does, they'll change channels). Art, life—who gives a shit?

Party of Dive: The Connors (Darlene—Sara Gilbert; Becky—Lecy Goranson, Sarah Chalke; D.J.—Michael Fishman)/*Roseanne*. D.J. is his father's son—in terms of his closet selection, the denim apple doesn't fall far from the flannel tree. The girls are a different story. Darlene Connor is the anti-Laura Ingalls—she wouldn't touch a sunbonnet with a ten-foot pool cue. "She's gone from being a tomboy in sport jerseys and beat-up jeans to an art-punk in head-to-toe black," says Quigley. "Basically, she'll wear anything that's comfortable, goes against the grain, and has a studied 'don't care' attitude." Most recently, Darlene toughs it out in antique shirts or funky Ts with altered vintage men's pleated pants, in a gamut of hues ranging from powder blue and gray to dark purple, green, rust, and olive. American Rag dresses her ragtag, down-home vintage side; Rage and Contempo Casuals dress her, um, angry, contemporary casual side. Funny how that works.

Be a *Roseanne*-ite—or just look like one.

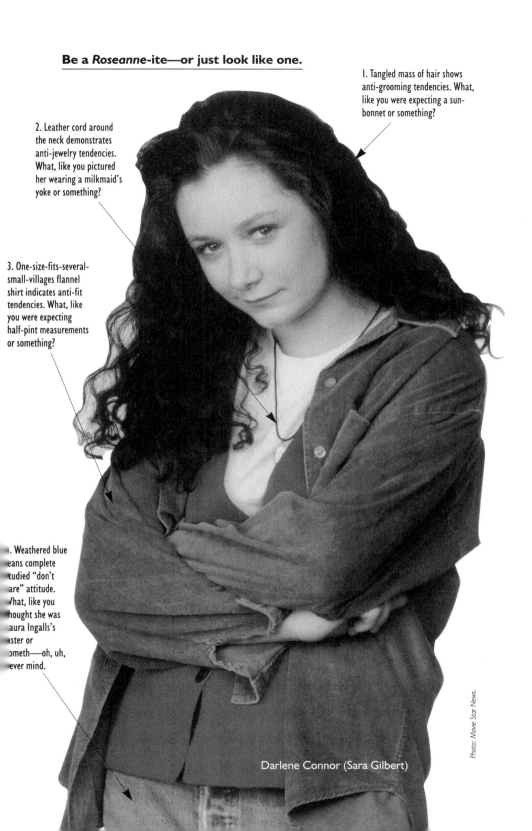

1. Tangled mass of hair shows anti-grooming tendencies. What, like you were expecting a sun-bonnet or something?

2. Leather cord around the neck demonstrates anti-jewelry tendencies. What, like you pictured her wearing a milkmaid's yoke or something?

3. One-size-fits-several-small-villages flannel shirt indicates anti-fit tendencies. What, like you were expecting half-pint measurements or something?

4. Weathered blue jeans complete studied "don't care" attitude. What, like you thought she was Laura Ingalls's sister or someth—oh, uh, never mind.

Darlene Connor (Sara Gilbert)

Photo: Movie Star News.

Regarding Becky—or rather, Beckys—the effect is softer and more feminine. Originally, Quigley kept the character in floral, lacy pastels, but when she got married and moved to a trailer park, "We let go of the Little Bo Peep thing." She still leans heavily on skirts and dresses with great success—one sundress with a denim bib and patchwork skirt sparked a national trend. After that, *everybody* wanted to live in a trailer park.

Party of Jive: The Bundys (Kelly—Christina Applegate; Bud—David Faustino). Say what you will about Al and Peg Bundy, they sure raised two trend-a-rific kids! At the tender age of fifteen, Kelly burst upon the scene in Spandex—and thousands of teenage boys across the country burst right along with her. Now in her mid-twenties, she's less tramp—which lamentably leaves her fans less damp. Squires shops for Kelly in many of the same stores that clothe *Melrose Place*. "She's up-to-the-minute," says Squires, "we keep a close eye on the current trends." Cropped tops, short skirts, and low-slung bell bottoms fill the bill, as do Levi's, halter tops, platform shoes, and lace-up combat boots. In a switch from her dog-collar and chain days, jewelry is scarce. With all that skin showing, who needs jewelry?

Brother Bud made the transition from nerd to grunge, and became an unexpected sex symbol to boot. There's no accounting for people's taste. Jeans, T-shirts, and sneakers are the grunge du jour; a stud earring and beaded necklaces are the final coup de grunge. As with most guys, department stores and GAP are his major fashion sources. And now that our little boy's a great big college man, he's not only Bud-older—he's Bud-wiser.

Party of Five: The Salingers (Charlie—Matthew Fox; Bailey—Scott Wolf; Julia—Neve Campbell; Claudia—Lacey Chabert; Owen—Andrew and Steven Cavarno). *Party* seems an odd word choice for the title of a show that's based on a bunch of

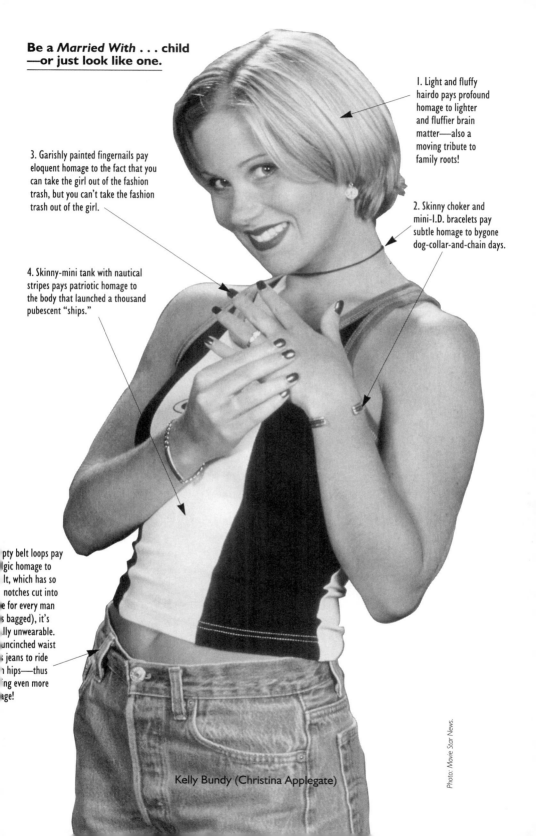

Be a *Married With* . . . child —or just look like one.

1. Light and fluffy hairdo pays profound homage to lighter and fluffier brain matter—also a moving tribute to family roots!

3. Garishly painted fingernails pay eloquent homage to the fact that you can take the girl out of the fashion trash, but you can't take the fashion trash out of the girl.

2. Skinny choker and mini-I.D. bracelets pay subtle homage to bygone dog-collar-and-chain days.

4. Skinny-mini tank with nautical stripes pays patriotic homage to the body that launched a thousand pubescent "ships."

pty belt loops pay gic homage to lt, which has so notches cut into e for every man s bagged), it's lly unwearable. uncinched waist s jeans to ride h hips—thus ng even more age!

Kelly Bundy (Christina Applegate)

Photo: Movie Star News.

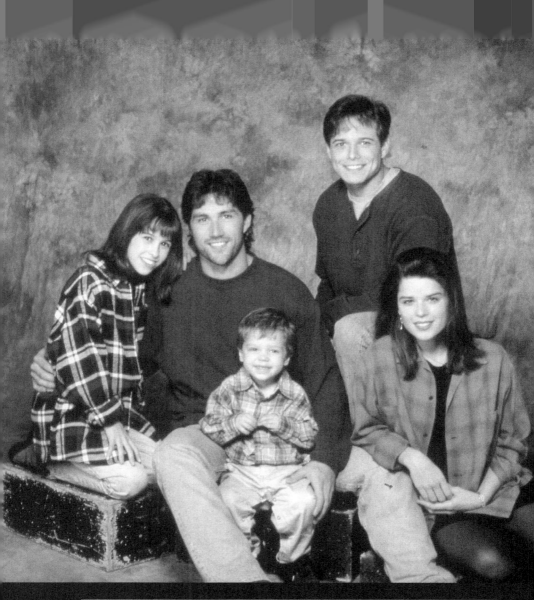

Their table is waiting. The Salinger family takes *Five* (as in *Party of*), clockwise from the pretty, perky adolescent on the left: Claudia (Lacey Chabert) is sweet, fleecy and most importantly, not in overalls; Charlie (Matthew Fox) holds the crew together in a quasi-rugged kind of way; Bailey (Scott Wolf) unbuttons a new collegiate look; Julia (Neve Campbell) stretches her dancer's legs; and baby Owen (Andrew or Steven Cavarno) is so nice, they kids' parents being killed in a car crash . . . but who are we to judge? After all, we're book people—*and this is television.*

In any case, this gang of five grew up and caught on fast—and so did their wardrobes. Oldest brother Charlie stays neat and comfortable (no grunge, please) in Levi's 501s or Banana Republic pants and flannel shirts with a T-shirt underneath. "He's supposed to look responsible, but he doesn't have time to do more than reach in his closet and throw on whatever's there," says costume designer Scilla Andreen-Hernandez. "I keep him in layers because the show's set in San Francisco, and it's cold there. Charlie has two sport coats for job interviews, both ill fitting—the idea being that his mother bought one of them a while back, and the other he got at a thrift store and never had tailored. When he's working at Salinger's (the family restaurant), he wears nice shirts, Banana Republic black twill pants, and the official Salinger's tie—teal and cream colored with columns that "look like Michelangelo's sketches," says Andreen-Hernandez. Charlie wears Red Wing boots and his only jewelry is a practical watch.

Younger brother Bailey is still in high school, and dresses accordingly. Overdyed black, brown, or blue Levi's, work boots and earth-toned long- and short-sleeved T-shirts from GAP or Calvin Klein make up most of his wardrobe. "If we can't find the color we want, we buy Hanes T-shirts and dye them ourselves," says Andreen-Hernandez. All of Bailey's clothes (and Charlie's, for that matter), are distressed for that well-worn feeling. "Nothing should look off the rack," Andreen-Hernandez says. "When I buy new jeans, I have the actor take them home and wear them so that they'll look broken-in on camera." Bailey's signature piece: a Verso car coat with black stitching, orange flannel lining, and a cord collar. "We get more calls on that coat," says Andreen-Hernandez. "Wolf is so handsome, he looks good in anything. We keep it simple because he can wear anything well."

On the sisterhood front, Julia graces the screen "in clothes that flow and move," says Andreen-Hernandez. "She's a dancer, and I like the way she glides when she walks." She avoids anything that's tucked in or buttoned down, opting instead for rayon skirts with boots, tight tops, and cropped sweaters in saturated tones. "Julia is comfortable, simple, and pared down; her clothes should hang well and look a little different from your typical high-schooler," says Andreen-Hernandez. But don't waste time hoping for a navel sighting—that's not her style. Ditto for pastels and brights. "When I don't buy Bisou Bisou or DKNY, I like to go to the old ladies' section of department stores, take a shirt, tint and distress it, cut it, and then have Julia wear it as a dress or blouse." Andreen-Hernandez isn't drawn to labels—they're too generic—so she goes to vintage stores. "I even hunt through my grandmother's closet. She's saved everything from the 1940s." Thank God for family.

This season, Claudia, the youngest girl, finally steps out of her overworn overalls. "She's an adolescent now," says Andreen-Hernandez. "She likes oversized shirts from the forties and fifties from American Rag or Rag Tattoo. We alter them and she wears them with leggings and jeans." F.Y.I.: Claudia will be wearing a bra this season, and Andreen-Hernandez anticipates rebellious times ahead. This will set the stage for lots of black clothes, combat boots, and "hard-looking stuff," says Andreen-Hernandez. "I'll keep patterns to a minimum and stick to solids."

And last but not least, Owen makes a bold fashion statement in crisp, white diapers. Luckily, he's a baby, so this works well for him. Before you know it, he'll be walking and talking, wearing long pants, and heading off to begin his **School Days**. Or as we like to call it, **Chapter 9**.

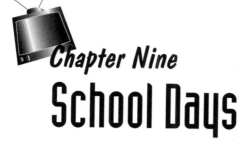

Chapter Nine

School Days

FRIDAY, 9:00 P.M. (ABC) CLUELESS

(1996–present). *Clueless* (the movie) comes to television. Wealthy, beautiful, exceedingly well dressed students in a Beverly Hills high school bop and shop with a social conscience. MTV top-twenty soundtrack.

SUNDAY, 8:30 P.M. (NBC) BOSTON COMMON

(1996–present). *Forrest Gump* (the inexplicable phenomenon) comes to television. Cash-poor, semi-beautiful, exceedingly dressed-down students in a Boston college drawl and y'all with a social conscience. TNN top-twenty soundtrack.

Good morning, students.

Our topic today is school on television. Network executives' interest in the educational experience was firmly established in the 1950s, when a hit series called—show of hands? anyone?—*Our Miss Brooks* captured the attention of viewers nationwide. Since then, small-screen classrooms have proliferated. We enjoyed inner-city adolescent high-jinks in *Welcome Back, Kotter,* a sitcom that launched the roller-coaster career of a popular movie actor named—anyone? anyone?—John Travolta. We studied law at Harvard University in—anyone? title of dramatic series about law school? anyone?—*The Paper Chase,* and watched with grim fascination as the teenage boarders on *The Fats of Life,* or rather *The Facts of Life* grew—larger or smaller? show of hands? anyone?—larger than actual life itself.

More recently, political causes and style trends fill the syllabus of *Beverly Hills, 90210,* a program about a group of earnest young people in—anyone? anyone?—Los Angeles.

This season brings us two new infusions of prime-time curricula. The first, *Clueless,* is based on the movie of the same name, and centers on the highly fashionable exploits of its heroine, named after a one-named singer in the seventies who makes infomercials—anyone? anyone?—Cher. The second, *Boston Common,* is appropriately set in—hazard a guess? anyone?—Boston, and concerns the fish-out-of-water adventures of Boyd Pritchett and his sister, Wyleen. In keeping with television tradition, clothing plays a major role in each; the tremendous attention to wardrobe is almost enough to make the rest of the show, well, academic. On that note, any questions? Anyone? Anyone? We'll be passing out your style report cards shortly. If you wish to discuss a grade, please wait to do so until the commercial break. Class dismissed.

Name: Cher (Rachel Blanchard) / *Clueless.*

Grade: A

Comments: Cher gets top marks for her knowledge of fashion alone. "She's the kind of girl who goes to Europe for the couture collections," says costume designer Mona May, "and then incorporates them into high-school-age looks." Her central style concept is simple sophistication, as seen through the eyes of a sixteen-year-old. A rich sixteen-year-old. With designers like Azzedine Alaia, Dolce & Gabanna, Jill Stuart, Vivienne Tam, and Calvin Klein populating her closet, she's clearly not buying her clothes with money she makes on some after-school paper route. In terms of fit, "Her clothes are always tight and short, never oversized," says May. "She's got a great stomach for hip-huggers." More frequently, she wears little A-line skirts and dresses, often with a cropped or hip-length jacket. Shiny Mary Janes may accent a dropped-waist dress (Cher doesn't wear heels), but her feet are the only place you'll see black. Rather, she goes for "cool colors like pink, blue, green, cream, light yellow, or white," says May. No earth tones, no jewel tones, and nowaynohow Birkenstocks. As if! She's light, bright, and breezy—without being overdone. "If anything, she's underdone," says May. Okeydoke. Her accessories enhance her outfits, but don't match exactly; for example, her teddy bear backpack should be a complementary color, rather than the same color as her dress. Baby barrettes, small purses, and fuzzy faux-fur collars fill the rest of her drawers. If it's cute, cuddly, and screechingly overpriced, she's all over it. Clueless? Yes. Penniless? Puh-lease.

Name: Dionne (Stacy Dash) / *Clueless*.

Grade: A-

Comments: Cher's best friend, Dionne, rates by getting down and being funky (the obvious teenage alternative to getting high and being a junkie). "She's a rich black girl in a rich white neighborhood," says May. "She knows French fashion, but she incorporates a black, Diana Ross feel to it." This is achieved by combining modern high-fashion with thrift-store stuff like vintage purses, micro-minis and big platform shoes from the sixties. "Dionne will show much more bare skin than Cher," says May. "She's hot and slick—within a high-school context." May plays up the hot-slick effect by using bright colors—mainly jewel tones, with some fuchsia, lime green, and neon yellows thrown in to add, uh, dash. Dionne also goes wild with Pucci-esque patterns—again, a sixties staple. Her designers of choice are Mark Wong Nark, Diesel, Vertigo, and Dolce & Gabbana. Her jewelry is "cool, hip, not too big," and exclusively gold—because silver's out of the question, and platinum would be, like, gauche.

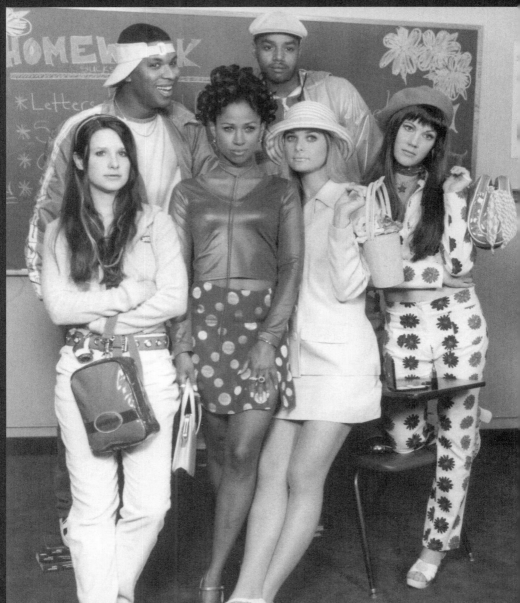

Scenes from a mall. The adorably adolescent cast of *Clueless* (left to right: Heather Gottlieb, Sean Holland, Stacy Dash, Donald Adeosun Faison, Rachel Blanchard, Elisa Donavan) displays timeless elegance and quiet dignity. As if!

Name: Joy Byrnes (Traylor Howard) /*Boston Common.*

Grade: A-

Comments: Joy is the very image of a graduate student/teaching assistant at a New England college. Luckily for her, she *is* a graduate student/teaching assistant at a New England college since it'd be a strange look for, say, a zookeeper. Her clothes come from accessible stores such as Banana Republic and J. Crew, with a few expensive pieces from Barneys on the side. "We want her to be elegant and cute," says costume designer Laurie Eskowitz. The actress is so petite, Eskowitz custom-makes many of her straight, cropped cigarette pants out of vintage fabrics, including old drapes, curtains, and tablecloths. And while she does do patterned pants, Joy generally sticks to solids—navy, brown, white, and beige, with a few touches of orange, red, and turquoise. Twin sets, lots of cardigans, clogs, leather zip-up ankle boots, and a little chiffon scarf tied around her neck complete the collegiate look (in *Melrose Place*, it's considered the Parisian look, but, hey, opposite coast).

Name: Murray (Donald Adeosun Faison) /*Clueless.*

Grade: B+

Comments: May describes Dionne's boyfriend, Murray, as "a hot, slick Beverly Hills boy" (evidently, there's a major flux of "hot" and "slick" on that show). Like Dionne, he adds a street influence to his designer garb. "He wears baggy, low-slung pants and sportswear from Fila and Nike," says May. "He's not exactly a homeboy on the street—it's more of a homeboy silhouette with really expensive clothes and bright colors like green, blue, and orange." His higher-end stuff is from Mecca, Virgo, Donna Karan, and Calvin Klein. And, of course, his signature piece is That Hat. "He wears old men's caps and golf hats in almost every scene," says May. His shoes are equally eye-catching—tennis sneakers, motorcross boots, and indecently bright orange Doc Martens. "Whatever Murray wears is the hippest and the latest," she says. Uh, doesn't she mean the hottest and the slickest?

Name: Wyleen Pritchett (Hedy Burress) / *Boston Common.*

Grade: B+

Comments: Described by Eskowitz as "my Fred Segal girl," Wyleen is a typical college freshman figuring out the sartorial ropes. After a brief stint of flannel shirts and cowboy boots, she's transformed herself into a hip-hugged, Hush Puppied, baby-T-ed trendoid. Nonetheless, she's such a good student of fashion, she manages not to look contrived. "The character threw herself into learning how to dress," says Eskowitz. "It was a natural choice to have her evolve this way." Also typical of a college freshman, Wyleen stays on the casual side. What's more, since she's always broke, she makes the most of everything she's got. And we don't mean just clothes.

Name: Boyd Pritchett (Anthony Clark) / *Boston Common.*

Grade: B

Comments: Boyd Pritchett, Harrington College's resident janitor/ handyman/Mr. Fix-it-and-break-it-again-as-soon-as-possible, hasn't evolved quite as successfully as his sister. His wardrobe carries a southern flavor (more farm than charm): gabardine shirts from the 1940s and '50s, flat-front dickeys, shark-skin work pants, and work boots. His one stab at assimilation is a Boston Red Sox T-shirt under his vintage shirts. Still, Boyd wears these wildly unfashionable outfits with aplomb. Make that two plombs. His extra-special-lucky garment is "Big Collar," a shirt that has (you'll never guess) a big collar. Eskowitz found it at Palace Costume, a warehouse in Los Angeles. "It's gabardine with a purple-and-gray Western pattern;

I put silver clips on the tips of the collar to make them look even bigger," she says. "Big Collar"—which has been on display at Planet Hollywood—is supposed to infuse Boyd with incredible confidence, and make him feel sexy and cool. Or hot. Or slick.

Name: Tasha King (Tasha Smith) / *Boston Common.*

Grade: B

Comments: The head of Harrington's student union, Tasha is Boyd's good, best buddy, filling the role of wisecracking sidekick with . . . three plombs. Her top half dazzles in bold colors such as purple, pink, orange, and salmon; her bottom half is covered by pants in darker shades (since she's usually behind the desk at the student union, we rarely see her legs anyway). She plays up her long, braided hair with tortoise-shell earrings. "We put her in big-heeled Beatles boots, pleated wide-legged or straight pants, tight, ribbed sweaters, and period blouses," says Eskowitz. Quite frankly, we would've rated Tasha higher, but the phrase "period blouses" kind of turned our stomachs.

Name: Jack Reed (Vincent Ventresca) / *Boston Common.*

Grade: B-

Comments: Jack Reed (last seen as Fun Bobby on *Friends*), is *Boston Common*'s resident stuffed shirt. As a professor of communications, he wants to look like an authority figure, and his small, round glasses and preppy wrappings facilitate his mission. "We put him in J. Crew sweater vests, Banana Republic flat-front khakis, and loafers," says Eskowitz. "His jackets are fairly straight, small in the shoulders, single-breasted, and have two or three buttons; his colors are conservative—navy, white, blue, and yellow." The only bold items in his closet are his ties, which are often a daring, daring red, with scandalous patterns like sailboats. The concept is very New England, very laced up, very conservative. "I want him to look like he used to row crew—which he did, in real life," says Eskowitz. So, would that be crew as in boats, or crew as in J.?

Name: Tai (Heather Gottlieb) / *Clueless.*

Grade: C+

Comments: Light-years behind the times, Tai persists in holding the banner of grunge aloft—and askew. "She's trying to learn from the other girls, but it's not working," says May. She forgoes designer labels completely, heading instead for trendy low-end stores like Contempo Casuals or vintage shops. Once there, she reliably chooses ill-fitting clothes in poor color combinations. "Sometimes she wears army clothes or surfer clothes," says May. "The overall look is supposed to be messy and uneven." We'll say. Unflattering hues, off-putting dyed fake hairpieces, and sloppy makeup wash her out further, thus making our young Tai . . . wan. (Sorry, we couldn't resist.)

Name: Leonard Prince (Steve Paymer) / *Boston Common.*

Grade: D

Comments: Across-the-hall neighbor Leonard Prince's clothes come in two colors: brown and gray. "Everything is pilled and old and one hundred percent cotton," says Eskowitz. A shoe archivist on the show, his decrepit sweaters and shabby tweed jackets with elbow patches are supposed to convey the image of an absentminded academe who spends too much time thinking about shoes and no time thinking about clothes (meanwhile, if he's spending so much time thinking about shoes, what's he doing wearing Wallabees?). His pants—flat-front polyester jobbies—are either very long or

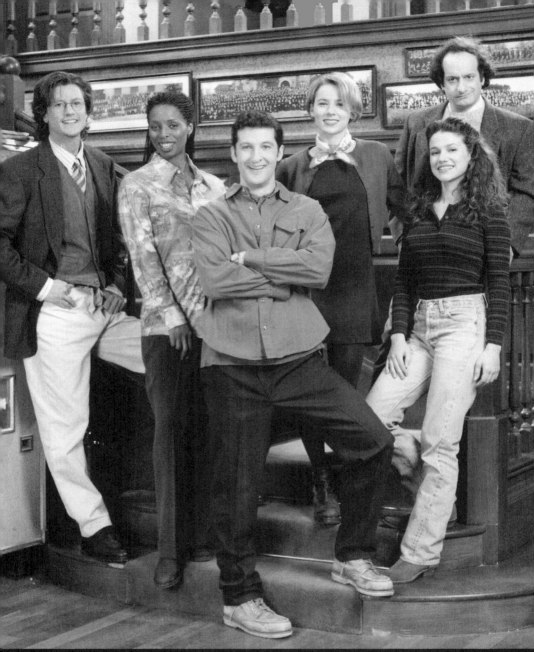

Boston Common is the big cast on campus. Starting from the preppie milque-
toast on left: Jack (Vincent Ventresca) is all ivy, no league; Tasha (Tasha Smith)
hits home plait; Boyd (Anthony Clark) steeps in Southern comfort; Joy
(Traylor Howard) makes us want to scarf; Leonard (Steve Paymer) is the next
worst thing to being naked; and Wyleen (Hedy Burress) needs a good belt.

too short. "He's your basic schlepp," says Eskowitz. Interesting aside: actor Steve Paymer was a writer for *Mad About You* and *The Single Guy* (his brother, David Paymer, was the ice cream mogul in *City Slickers*). *Boston Common*'s producers created the character for him—and patterned the character's wardrobe after the actor's own. Ouch. Mind you, his clothing is by no means indicative of all writers. Like, if someone created sitcom characters based on us, they'd be really, really well dressed.

Name: Amber (Elisa Donovan) / *Clueless*.

Grade: D-

Comments: *Quelle* mess. "Amber takes trends too literally," says May. "If she's wearing something, it's a sign that you shouldn't." In other words, before you lay out a bunch of cash for a rubber pant suit or an Astroturf skirt, you might want to reconsider. "Sometimes we dress her in themes, like the Eskimo outfit with a fake-fur jacket and boots," says May. Pippi Longstocking, the Jetsons, and beat poets are other sources of inspiration; Lacroix and Moschino top the designer list. The reigning accessories queen, Amber matches everything with painstaking precision. "Once we put her in rain gear," May recalls. "She was plastic from head to toe, including her purse and galoshes." The trick with this character: mixing tons of pieces to create the ultimate fashion victim. A couture casualty. This chick needs intensive care. Someone call a doctor! Rush her to the ER! Quick, while there's still Hope! (Can you see where we're going here? **Chapter 10**, of course. **Doctors' Orders**.)

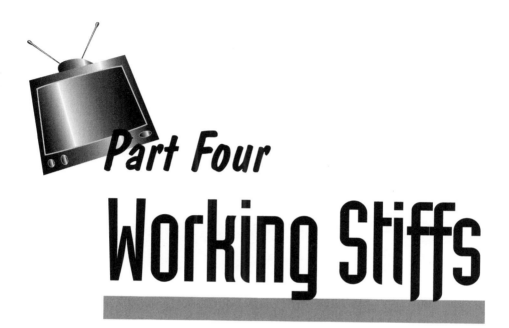

Part Four

Working Stiffs

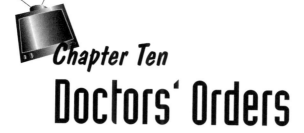

Chapter Ten
Doctors' Orders

THURSDAY, 10:00 P.M. (NBC) ER

(1994–present). Gripping hospital drama centered around emergency room in Chicago's County General Memorial Hospital. Talented ensemble-cast grapples with life-and-death epiphanies, as well as ways to get blood-stains out of various colored scrubs. Personal dilemmas galore; patchwork surgery. Serious adrenaline transfusion via the tube. Tune in—stat.

MONDAY, 10:00 P.M. (CBS) CHICAGO HOPE

(1994–present). Gripping hospital drama centered around neurosurgeon and colleagues in Chicago Hope Hospital. Talented ensemble-cast grapples with life-and-death epiphanies, as well as ways to get blood-stains out of custom-made operating caps. Ethical dilemmas galore; state-of-the-art surgery. Moderate adrenaline transfusion via the tube. Please tune in—stat.

TUESDAY, 9:00 P.M. (NBC) FRASIER

(1993–present). Nipping psychological sitcom centered around call-in radio psychoanalyst and his family in Seattle. Talented ensemble-cast grapples with each other, as well as ways to get blue-blood stains out of Armani suits. Hypothetical dilemmas galore—pedantic surgery of the English language. Reasonable nitrous oxide transfusion via the tube. Do try to tune in—whenever it's convenient.

Maestro, some lush orchestral accompaniment, please.

Maladies . . .
In the corners of our eyes,
Gritty, technicolored maladies,
Of the way ER.

Shattered pictures,
Of the bile we left behind,
Bile we gave to Hope and Frasier,
And the way ER.

La, la, la-dee—oh, sorry, we didn't hear you come in. What seems to be the problem? Does it hurt when you do that? Then keep doing it until we can get a plot line going.

Which shouldn't take too long. Ever since the days of Ben Casey, maladies have kept the networks humming. Showgirl with a hemorrhoid? Get Dr. Ross for some smooth operating—*stat!* Christian Scientist with a hangnail? Page Dr. Austin for an anguished ethical dilemma—*stat!* Plumber with water on the brain? Call Dr. Crane for a towel—*splat!* Whether it's hammertoes or sickle-cell anemia, before you can say, *and while you're at it, hurry up,* you'll be whisked on a long day's gurney into night.

Of course, all wounds need dressing, and these shows are no exception. Would you trust an ungloved surgeon or an unwrapped shrink? We say no. TV being a highly visual medium (or hadn't you noticed?), a doctor's garb is crucial in conveying his or her specialty, bedside manner, and overall personality. It's one of the few places where John Weitz has more clout than Johns Hopkins.

The most critical element on the sartorial triage list: scrubs. Without question, they comprise the bulk of both *ER*'s and *Chicago Hope*'s wardrobes (granted, they don't show up on *Frasier*, but since that's only a half hour, and *ER* and *CH* are each a full hour, we figure they outnumber *Frasier*, four to one). These snazzy little outfits demand more effort than you might think. Because they're not just the human equivalent of lobster bibs, you know. *They're a matter of life or death.* As such:

Rules for Customary Scrub Procedure:

Procedure A:

Since *ER* is primarily set in the, er, ER, the characters practically live in scrubs—and correspondingly, the scrubs look lived in. According to Lynn Paolo, costume designer for ER, "We distress the scrubs and lab coats by washing them a hundred times." In the ER, they're dyed a pleasing shade of green for your viewing pleasure; in the operating room or, er, the OR, blue becomes the regulation shade. After a two-year period of trial and error, the nurses are currently wearing rose. "We started out with peach, but it wasn't flattering on Julianna Margulies," says Paolo. "When we switched to burgundy, the producers said everyone looked too good because you couldn't see the blood. So then we went to teal—but that wasn't right because it was too close to the blue of the surgeons' scrubs. Finally, we settled on rose—it's flattering, you can see the blood, and it doesn't conflict with other colors." Holy moly—this medicine is a tough business.

Outside the confines of the emergency room, the color wheel is still your best compass. "When we first started the show, [creator]

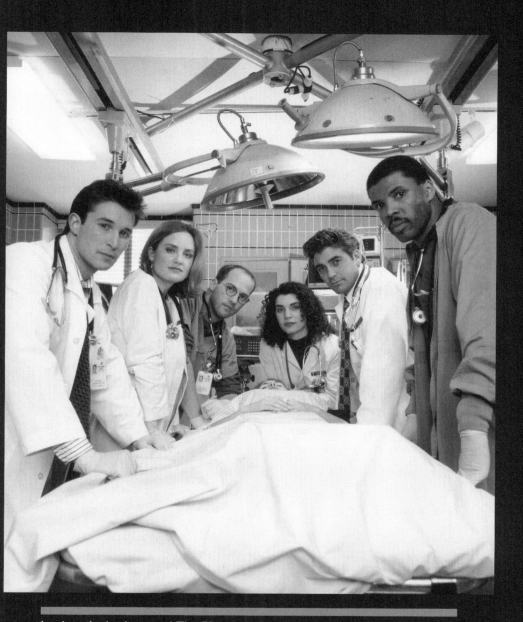

Look at the birdie—stat! The *ER* cast strikes a pose while the woman on the table languishes . . . patiently? Starting from the hottie-doc on the left: Dr. Carter (Noah Wyle) looks impish in a lab coat; Dr. Lewis (Sherry Stringfield) looks contemplative in a lab coat; Dr. Greene (Anthony Edwards) looks concerned in scrubs; Nurse Hathaway (Julianna Margulies) looks sexy in a lab coat; Dr. Ross (George Clooney) looks dreamy in a lab coat; and Dr. Benton (Eriq LaSalle) looks angry in scrubs. Clearly, scrubs are a major personality downer.

Michael Crichton said we should know what someone does by the color of their scrubs," recalls Paolo. When Crichton talks, wardrobe listens. Accordingly, doctors in oncology wear bright blue and hot pink scrubs (to cheer up patients), ob/gyn residents wear pink and baby blue (to program infant minds with gender stereotypes from the get-go), and pediatricians in the children's intensive care unit wear light blue (to show off George Clooney's dreamy eyes). Occasionally, Paolo does mix things up: Carter sometimes wears caps with different patterns—like the reindeer cap he wore on a Christmas episode—and Hicks has one with an African pattern. On the whole, though, this is not a major venue for humorous style statements. That's what *Friends* is for.

As for the "standard" white cotton lab coats, "Greene and Weaver wear full-length lab coats," says Paolo. "Med students are supposed to wear shorter ones, but we put Carter in full-length because he was a cocky kid. In a real hospital, he would've been forced to change." Wait, what do you mean *real* hospital? Originally, the coats were a cotton-polyester blend. "We like to put light layers under the scrubs and coats to show that it's cold in Chicago, but the poly-blend was too hot for the actors." Now, in addition to being 100 percent cotton, the lab coats are also all custom-designed. Doctor's orders, we guess.

Procedure B:

Unlike its main rival, *Chicago Hope* is set in a top-of-the-line private hospital—and this difference is telegraphed by the condition of the scrubs. "We never distress our scrubs or lab coats," says Brad Loman, the show's costume designer. "We want them to look crisp, clean, and bright. The [all cotton] lab coats should be white and pristine." In the ER and OR, cornflower blue scrubs are the rule; beyond these areas, the hospital is, again, color-coded. "Pediatrics is pink," says Loman. "Infectious diseases is yellow, obstetrics is purple, and neurology is dark blue." (So, like, if you mixed a pediatrician with a neurologist, does that mean you'd get an obstetrician?) Loman also experiments with patterned caps, but only on Christine Lahti's Dr. Kate Austin. "I bought the fabric—it's an olive, rust, gold, and black paisley floral design—and we make the caps ourselves. They add to her individuality and character. Plus, the colors are flattering on her." Adam Arkin's Dr. Aaron Shutt wears an immaculately pressed lab coat most of the time. "He's a neurosurgeon and he goes on rounds to see patients," says Loman. "We want him to look professional, and the lab coat does it." Are you listening, all you medical students out there? Forget those silly textbooks and charts—buy an iron!

Mind you, doctors cannot live in scrubs alone. Below, a case-by-case study of our M.D.'s and their fashion M.O.'s, categorized by their prevailing plot ailments. Doctors, heel thyselves.

HEART DEFICIENCIES

Greenetic Displacement

Identifying characteristics: Dr. Mark Greene (Anthony Edwards)/*ER.*

Symptoms: Utter immersion in work as a distraction from emotional anguish.

Causes: Abandonment by cheating wife, ensuing custody battle for daughter.

Diagnostic techniques: Psychological screening for paternal tendencies, preliminary closet examination for signs of fashion apathy.

Treatment: Simple as can be. Character should follow a regimen of "clothes with a lived-in look"—soft cords, T-shirts, V-neck sweaters, and pants from stores like Eddie Bauer and GAP. "We're going for a dad look on him," explains Paolo. Giant down coats are prescribed for warmth, Nikes or hiking boots for comfort, and round wire glasses for "surprise sex symbol" effect.

Lewisterectomy

Identifying characteristics: Dr. Susan Lewis (Sherry Stringfield)/*ER*.

Symptoms: Utter immersion in work to discover greater meaning of life.

Causes: Court order to relinquish Baby Susie to former-alcoholic sister.

Diagnostic techniques: Careful monitoring of paycheck deposit stubs for confirmation that character makes sufficient money to maintain upscale image.

Treatment: Conservative—pleated trousers, blouses, and suits of the Calvin Klein and Donna Karan variety. Colors range from lemon and pink to chocolate and navy. To alleviate discomfort due to chronic standing, low-impact shoes (such as penny loafers, clogs, or sneakers) are mandatory. Jewelry should be limited to tiny doses of silver. "We do put Sherry in some funny winter hats and big bulky winter coats with mittens," says Paolo. Upon hospital release, character may benefit from T-shirts, men's drawstring pajama bottoms— and a great big doll named Susie!

Sub-acute Shuttosis

Identifying characteristics: Dr. Aaron Shutt (Adam Arkin)/*CH*.

Symptoms: Utter immersion in work to facilitate denial and depression.

Causes: Wife sleeping with younger doctor.

Diagnostic techniques: Acid test for character's potential to become less acerbic, thereby demonstrating a more sympathetic, if still nervous, system.

Treatment: In flux. Initial experiments with Armani and Valentino single-breasted crepe suits and designer ties proved successful, but engendered an undesirable side effect of stuffiness. To counterbalance this, an increase in slacks, vests, and three-button sport coats may be required. "We want to make him more huggable," explains Loman. "He's the sweetest guy in the world, and this moves him into the comfort zone." In addition, a softening of the palette (to browns, olives, taupes, and warm charcoals) has had promising results. Final measures include Rockport Dress-port shoes and Prozac emotional sup-port tablets.

Crane's Syndrome (Frasier strain)

Identifying characteristics: Dr. Frasier Crane (Kelsey Grammer)/*Frasier*.

Symptoms: Utter immersion in unlikely living situation with erudite younger brother and implausibly redneck father in order to create spin-off of wildly popular sitcom set in Boston bar.

Causes: Adulteress wife gains custody of child, declines role on spin-off.

Diagnostic techniques: Blue-blood work and social X rays for evidence of innate ability to remain charming and witty in any situation.

Treatment. Multilevel. "Frasier isn't a trendy dresser, but he wants to look smart," says Audrey Bansmer, the show's costume designer. To add dimension, Bansmer prescribes layers of texture and rich color in monochromatic form. "The layers work for a couple reasons," says Bansmer. "I usually have to move Frasier from his home to the radio station. His home is light, so he has to wear dark clothes. The station is dark, so he has to wear light. This means he'll leave his house wearing a dark jacket, and then take off the jacket at the sta-

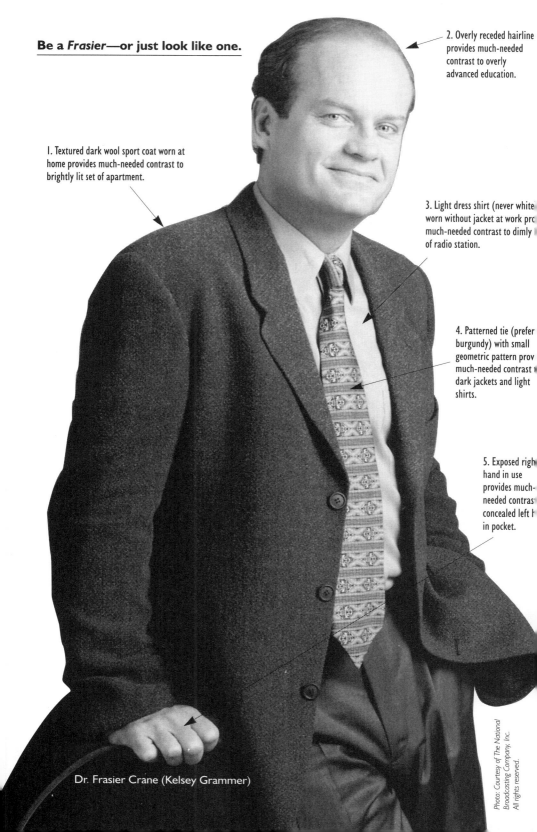

Be a *Frasier*—or just look like one.

1. Textured dark wool sport coat worn at home provides much-needed contrast to brightly lit set of apartment.

2. Overly receded hairline provides much-needed contrast to overly advanced education.

3. Light dress shirt (never white) worn without jacket at work pro much-needed contrast to dimly of radio station.

4. Patterned tie (prefer burgundy) with small geometric pattern prov much-needed contrast dark jackets and light shirts.

5. Exposed righ hand in use provides much- needed contras concealed left h in pocket.

Dr. Frasier Crane (Kelsey Grammer)

tion to show a light shirt underneath." Note that white shirts are never administered; olive, navy, or burgundy are the preferred substitutes, followed by a patterned sweater-vest or a six- or seven-button wool vest or waistcoat for a vintage-contemporary effect. Eighty percent of ties should be burgundy with small geometric patterns, and partially obscured by a wool or tweed sport coat, and an overcoat from Armani or Donna Karan. Frequency of suits should be minimal; pleated trousers and traditional lace-up wingtips are encouraged. Radio-station training optional.

Crane's Syndrome (Niles strain)

Identifying characteristics: Dr. Niles Crane (David Hyde Pierce)/*Frasier.*

Symptoms: Utter immersion in unlikely living situation with erudite older brother and implausibly redneck father in order to increase spin-off's chances of success.

Causes: Shrill wife berates character into leaving her.

Diagnostic techniques: Blue-blood work and social X rays for evidence of innate ability to sustain impeccable enunciation in any situation.

Treatment: Radically traditional. "Niles is more conservative than Frasier," says Bansmer. "He always wears double-breasted suits with suspenders to make him appear more powerful." Within this conservative framework, current trends should be applied liberally: e.g., designers such as Hugo Boss and Donna Karan, adventurous colors such as deep teal blue or eggplant, along with more standard browns, blues, and grays. Ties are bold and colorful with unique prints, and a high occurrence of Armani. Shirts are always striped. In the event that character indicates a desire to be more casual, jacket removal is permitted, but only when absolutely necessary.

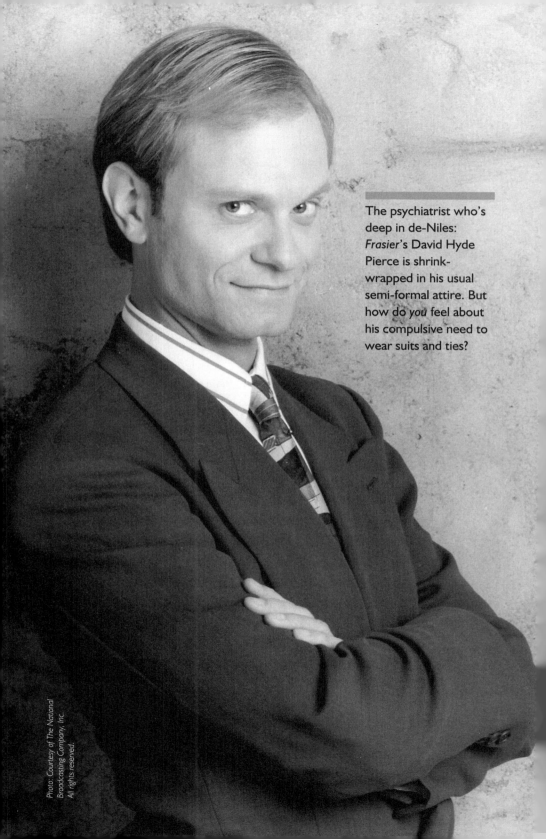

The psychiatrist who's deep in de-Niles: *Frasier*'s David Hyde Pierce is shrink-wrapped in his usual semi-formal attire. But how do *you* feel about his compulsive need to wear suits and ties?

HEART PALPITATIONS

Rosspiratory Distress
Identifying characteristics: Dr. Doug Ross (George Clooney)/*ER.*
Symptoms: Intense preoccupation with sub-sterling women, highly
infectious Caesar haircut.
Causes: Absent father leaves psychological void.
Diagnostic techniques: A standard MRI for indications that Inner-
Actor has requested his character be less playboyish, more
intense about his job.
Treatment: Repetitive. A steady recurrence of the same clothing
should emphasize plot-point of financial difficulties.
Nonetheless, while quantity of treatment is fairly low, quality
must remain high. Textured, tweedy jackets in somber colors (particularly dark brown), white or blue shirts, flat-front
pants, and Nike or Reebok sneakers should compensate for
earlier hot flashes of Casanova style. Character's seeming
lack of body flaws eliminates need for visual "bulk-up"
(through the use of sweaters, vests, or long-sleeved shirts
under scrubs); light T-shirts are sufficient. Hair should be
trimmed three times monthly.

Carter Tunnel Syndrome
Identifying characteristics: Dr. John Carter (Noah Wyle)/*ER.*
Symptoms: Intense preoccupation with self, highly infectious puppy-
dog demeanor.
Causes: Well-to-do family provides character with best of everything.
Diagnostic techniques: DNA scans for signs of acute entitlement,
and a romantic nature offset by narcissistic leanings.
Treatment: Developmental. Although the pre–medical school grad-
uation stage can be handled with preppy Brooks Brothers
suits and button-down shirts, as the condition matures, a

more sophisticated approach should be implemented, consisting of Hugo Boss and Armani suits with conservative blue or striped shirts. In both cases, Rockports are suggested for ambulatory support. Since the character's privileged background often causes him to have empathic difficulties, muted colors, soft sweaters, and suspenders can be helpful in maintaining an air of likability. (Warning: Suspenders that bear patterns depicting large-breasted women and other humorous images may not be visible to the viewer's eye.) Furthermore, the character's thin, long-waisted body-type may require visual "bulk-up" (see Treatments, Rosspiratory Distress), although primary hair care is considerably less vigilant.

Neo-Nyland infections

Identifying characteristics: Dr. Thomas Nyland (Thomas Gibson)/*CH*.

Symptoms: Intense preoccupation with alcohol, highly infectious schoolboy charm.

Causes: Compulsive need to hide fact of impoverished childhood. Oh, and alcohol.

Diagnostic techniques: Extensive psychotherapy for manifestations of a deep-seated Keeping-up-with-the-Welbys complex.

Treatment: Intentionally misleading. "He pretended to be from money, but really grew up poor," says Loman. "So when he's not in scrubs, he dresses in Ivy League–ish cashmere sweaters, button-down shirts, and dress slacks with blazers." Jewel tones like emerald, navy, and burgundy, and traditional Oxfords can further propagate the myth, in conjuction with a recommended daily allowance of Vitamin wanna-B$_2$.

Kronkitis

Identifying characteristics: Dr. Billy Kronk (Peter Berg)/*CH*.

Symptoms: Intense preoccupation with the principle of the thing, highly infectious surly charisma.

Causes: Feverish belief in medicine for the sake of medicine itself.

Diagnostic techniques: Stool sample examination to trace source of uncompromising moral fiber.

Treatment: Unpretentious and fiercely unassuming. A steady diet of brown leather jackets, jeans, well-washed flat-front khakis, T-shirts (by J. Crew, Calvin Klein, or Ralph Lauren's RRL line), flannel shirts, and shabby tweed sport coats is a potent method of conveying disdain for material pursuits. "Kronk doesn't care about image or money—he just cares about being a good doctor," says Loman. "And he wants a look that doesn't advertise what he does." In keeping with other related *CH* ailments, the favored palette is gray, olive, taupe, blue, brown, and black. Keep in mind that the character's unexpected departure from Rockports is not cause for alarm: an application of work boots will generally soothe his haggard individualism, although his condition will remain relentlessly critical.

Grad Mal Seizures

Identifying characteristics: Dr. Diane Grad (Jayne Brook) / *CH.*

Symptoms: Intense preoccupation with primates; infectious disease expertise.

Causes: Sudden realization that maybe an animal *lover* shouldn't be an animal *research doctor.*

Diagnostic techniques: Rehabilitative trip to Africa followed by a sudden, unexpected attack of galloping Kronkitis.

Treatment: Dangerously potent. The strength of Grad Mal's grip is powerful, and should not be ignored—particularly by those susceptible to Kronkitis. Effortless chic should be sustained through long and short skirts by Banana Republic or DKNY, short sweaters and vests in jewel tones (namely green) or buttery colors, tight pants, and full trousers. A stacked-heel loafer from Donna Karan or Charles David will provide additional style reinforcement. Under no circumstances should character be exposed to fur coats.

HEART BLOCKAGE

Benton-out-of-shape Disease

Identifying characteristics: Dr. Peter Benton (Eriq LaSalle)/*ER*.

Symptoms: Antisocial behavior accompanied by chronic head shaking.

Causes: A dearth of interpersonal skills, due to an overwhelming need to always be right.

Diagnostic techniques: Shoulder exam to locate chip.

Treatment: Isolated. Character should spend most of his time in blue scrubs to emphasize unhealthy obsession with work and magnify alienation. Because aftereffects of surgery yield a generous paycheck, non-scrub apparel can be more expensive—usually gray, brown, or black Armani and Calvin Klein suits over black T-shirts. Follow-up includes a black leather jacket and a gold-hoop or diamond-stud earring. Pierced ear may be emblematic of gaping holes in social life.

Austin-Barr Syndrome

Identifying characteristics: Dr. Kate Austin (Christine Lahti)/*CH*.

Symptoms: Antisocial behavior accompanied by chronic lip biting.

Causes: All-consuming position as head of surgery, semi-consuming battle with evil ex-husband for sole custody of child.

Diagnostic techniques: Shoulder examination to locate weight of entire world.

Treatment: Controlled. At least half of all clothing should be custom-designed, in the form of straight skirts, slacks, and a proliferation of fitted, single-breasted jackets. Application should

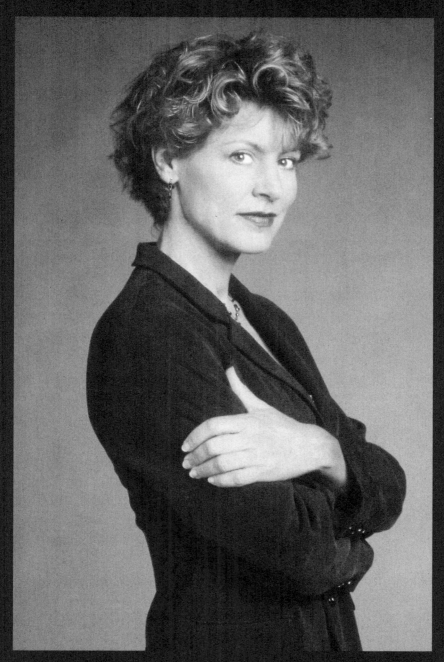

If you can see the chip on her shoulder, then YOU'RE TOO CLOSE. *Chicago Hope*'s Dr. Kathryn Austin (Christine Lahti) goes the distance by walking softly and carrying a big scalpel.

be clean, businesslike but accessible—and never fancy. Original designs may be alternated with designers like Jil Sander, Calvin Klein, and Armani. Nubbly silk, textured wools, and earth tones can offer prophylactic measures against inordinate uptightness. "She's got great legs, a muscular body, and a flat tummy, so you can't go wrong with her," says Loman. "For even more height, she wears a Donna Karan stacked-heel loafer." Lariat necklaces and other delicate antiquey earrings are acceptable. Caution: Lip rings could lead to excessive bleeding.

Finally, while in real life, doctors may think they're the only ones who matter, on TV they know better. Would that life could imitate art every now and then. Here, some of the most crucial support systems:

Nurse Carol Hathaway (Julianna Margulies)/*ER.*

Function: Cohesion. After attempting suicide in the very first episode, Nurse Hathaway realized anew the importance of life, and now serves as a moral compass for the rest of the cast.

Form: "She's a no-nonsense kind of girl," says Paolo. "We keep her in pants—Calvin Klein jeans, cords—and often oversized sweaters." Hathaway is decidedly working class, so she's rarely dressed up. "I don't want her to look like she's making an effort—high style isn't important to her," says Paolo. Low style suits her fine, especially those tailored scrubs that enhance her shapely figure. Her one indulgence is jewelry—delicate gemstone earrings set in gold, and dainty necklaces. "Julianna gets so excited when I bring in a new pair of earrings," says Paolo. "Wearing the jewelry helps her appear more feminine." The pre-Raphaelite ringlets don't hurt, either. Hey, just because you're moral doesn't mean you can't look pretty.

Efficiency rating (on a scale of 1 to 10): 8. We would've given her higher, except she caused that big ruckus about the color of the nurses' scrubs. Also, this adherence to morality stuff can really slow things down.

Dr. Phillip Watters (Hector Elizondo) / *CH.*

Function: Administration. Although a medical doctor in his own right, Watters's position as hospital administrator puts him on the business side of health. His judiciousness and political savvy keep *Chicago Hope* in the pink.

Form: In keeping with his duties, Watters sports a more corporate look. "We put him in single-breasted suits by Donna Karan, Calvin Klein, and Armani," says Loman. "Underneath, we go with crisp white shirts or pinstripes. He's worn tab collars, but we're moving away from that now." And in keeping with the rest of the cast, he wears—what else?—Rockports.

Efficiency rating: 10. Let's face it—Hector Elizondo is boss. We defy you to call him inefficient: the guy put Julia Roberts together in *Pretty Woman* with just one phone call—and it took Lyle Lovett over a year to dismantle her.

Daphne Moon (Jane Leeves) / *Frasier.*

Function: Physical therapy for the Cranes' father, visual therapy for the viewer.

Form: Eccentric—both in manner and clothing. "We started her out as a quirky thrift-store dresser," says Bansmer. "We made her clueless about color, mixing two blues that didn't go together, for example." When the character became Niles's love interest, however, Bansmer got more contemporary. "Now Daphne's the kind of woman who shops at Judy's or Contempo Casuals," says Bansmer. "The trendy clothes—cropped sweaters, baby T-shirts, little plaid or denim skirts, floral-print dresses—make her feel cute. Plus, she has an

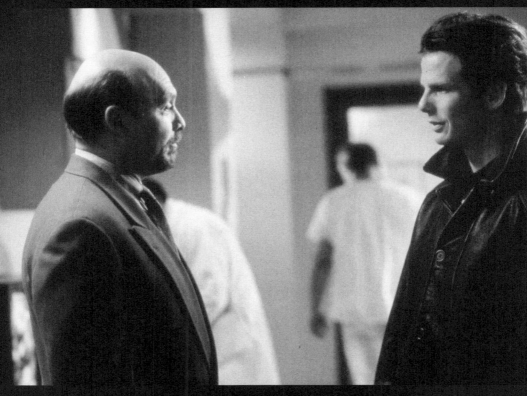

Pretty doctor, walking down the hall; pretty doctor, gosh he looks so tall. *Chicago Hope*'s Dr. Billy Kronk (Peter Berg, right) gets the once-over from hospital administrator Dr. Phillip Watters (Hector Elizondo).

Audrey Hepburn quality, so Capri pants look great on her." Her original quirkiness lives on, however, in her jewelry and accessories. She has a huge collection of thrift-store enamel and plastic pins, a 1940s-style purse made out of curtains, huge tote bags, high lace-up boots, and velvet slippers.

Efficiency rating: 7—She's a mite too scattered to focus entirely on any one thing. The woman's a psychic, a dancer, *Seinfeld*'s virgin, Miles Silverberg's ex-girlfriend, a floor wax, a dessert topping, and, oh yeah, a physical therapist. We need roller skates to keep up with her!

Roz Doyle (Peri Gilpin)/*Frasier.*

Function: Radio-show production, visual contrast to Daphne.

Form: Frasier's radio-show producer, Roz, is the antithesis of Daphne's girlishness. "She's a professional," says Bansmer. "She has nice clothes, but not a lot of them." Quality is key: well-tailored trousers, silk shirts, and fitted jackets—usually in black or brown with a bright piece thrown in. Like most working women, she mixes her separates in different combinations for different looks. "She has one pair of Donna Karan pants that she wears with everything, from a T-shirt, to a silk blouse, to a jacket," says Bansmer. You'll never see her in pastels or floral patterns. Even her jewelry is subtle— silver hoops and the occasional small pin. No slippers or boots on her, she sticks to TV–friendly stacked-heel loafers.

Efficiency rating: 9½ for being able to put on a radio show and star in a TV show at the same time. But how do *you* feel about her efficiency rating? *We're listening. . . .*

And that wraps up the medical portion of our program. We'll be back shortly with more footage of late-breaking events **In the News**—tune in at **11.**

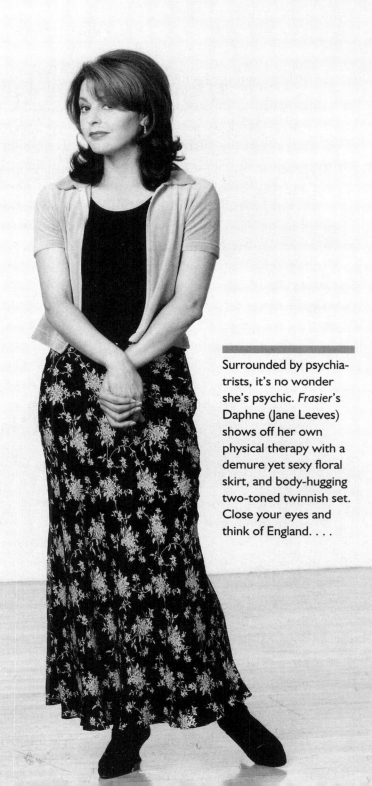

Surrounded by psychia-
trists, it's no wonder
she's psychic. *Frasier*'s
Daphne (Jane Leeves)
shows off her own
physical therapy with a
demure yet sexy floral
skirt, and body-hugging
two-toned twinnish set.
Close your eyes and
think of England. . . .

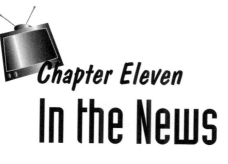

Chapter Eleven

In the News

Monday, 9:00 P.M. (CBS) MURPHY BROWN

(1988–present)

Dateline: Washington, D.C. Hemline: Knee high. Anchors at a prime-time news magazine trade barbs, sentiment, color rinse, and DKNY shoes. Front-page comedy and fashion.

Wednesday, 9:00 P.M. (NBC) NEWSRADIO

(1995–present).

Dateline: New York City. Hemline: Thigh high. Eclectic staff of a news radio station plays pranks, pulls fast ones, and lives for casual Mondays through Fridays. Static-free humor and wardrobe.

Tuesday, 9:30 P.M. (ABC) SPIN CITY

(1996–present).

Dateline: New York City. Hemline: Cuffed. Deputy mayor spins dirty laundry and sexual politics at City Hall, and nearly hangs himself by his power tie. Polls promising, but viewer votes not yet tabulated.

SUNDAY, 8:00 P.M. (ABC) LOIS AND CLARK: THE NEW ADVENTURES OF SUPERMAN

(1993–present).

Dateline: Gotham City. Hemline: Ankle to above the knee. Two reporters (and one alter ego) leap tall buildings, battle villains, and suit up in Calvin Klein. Above-the-fold romance and adventure.

THURSDAY, 9:30 P.M. (NBC) SUDDENLY SUSAN

(1996–present).

Dateline: San Francisco, California. Hemline: Flared. Lifestyle magazine editor searches for new identity, romance, and an on-the-record fashion statement. Subscriptions strong, but newsstand returns pending.

TO BE ANNOUNCED (NBC) THE NAKED TRUTH

(1995–present).

Dateline: Los Angeles, California. Hemline: Tea length (as in Tea Leoni). Magazine photojournalist pursues stories, sex life, and period pieces from thrift stores. Vintage jokes and style.

Prime Time Is Primed for News

THE MEDIA IS THE MESSAGE

Programs About News Industry
Flood Television Airwaves

By PHIL N. DEBLANK

TVLAND, 1996–97 Season—A quantitative survey of this season's television programs revealed today that an unprecedented one out of six situation comedies currently in production deals with media-related subject matter. While in the past, viewers tuned into a scattering of journalistic shows such as *Lou Grant* and *WKRP in Cincinnati,* this year, the genre has proliferated.

"Increasingly, the people who create TV have limited life experience outside their profession," said Rick Marin, television critic for *Newsweek* magazine. "What you're seeing is a generation of TV writers whose entire point of reference is the media. They write about what they know—and they end up creating shows about what they, or their friends, do."

Experts also cite the public's greater knowledge of the news-making industry as cause for the recent upsurgence. "These days, audiences are more savvy," said Marin. "Most viewers are aware of what the top ten programs are, how the ratings system works, or what the buzz is on new shows. Information that ten years ago would have been accessible only to industry insiders is now available everywhere. The public is fascinated with the media, the media provides more fuel for their fascination, and the whole thing feeds into itself."

To be sure, the television-generated perception of the

press bears only hazy resemblance to reality. For instance, the fall pilot of *Ink* depicted a newspaper reporter who wore a fedora and typed on an IBM Selectric—hardly the tools of a modern-day writer.

"The very idea of a fedora is an outrage," said Perry White, editor-in-chief of *The Daily Planet*. "It's an insult to the thousands of self-respecting fictional journalists who spend their fictional hard-earned money on designer suits, European jackets, custom-made unitards and red capes." White declined to comment on allegations that board member Calvin Klein was exploiting his position of power in an attempt to (*continued on Page C17, Column 3*)

And so it goes. Incidentally, if you're about to start searching for page C17, column 3, don't bother, because it doesn't exist. Or did you forget? *This is a book about television.* What's more, this is a chapter about news-related sitcoms on television, in a book about television. Below, a look at all the news-related fashion that's fit to print, in a chapter about news-related sitcoms on television, in a book (*continued on Page from Hell*)

LEAD STORY

Headliner: Murphy Brown (Candice Bergen)/*Murphy Brown*.

Capsule summary: An elegant Sprint (get it? get it?) to the finish.

Body copy: Back when Amanda Woodward was still T. J. Hookering (the T. J. being optional), Murphy Brown was already redefining the work-wear force. Bill Hargate, the show's sole costume designer, created Murphy's clean, relaxed office line, and women across the country followed suit—as well as slacks, jackets, and other mix-and-match separates. On the whole, Hargate prefers to stick with "the classics," and generally buys American. "We do a lot of Donna Karan, Calvin

Murphy's Law: Look before you quantum leap; don't speak at decibel levels lower than a fire alarm's—and never let 'em see your neck.

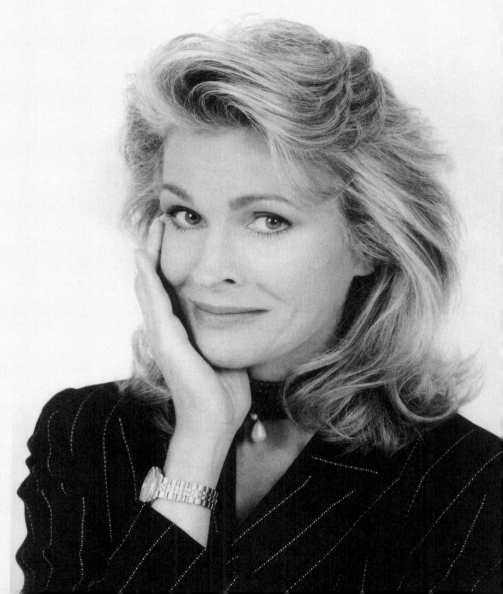

Klein and Ralph Lauren," says Hargate, "but the show's been on so long, I don't think there's any designer we haven't tried." Although he's experimented with a wide range of colors and fabrics, "camels and flannels" ultimately rate highest, with some blues, reds, golds, and yellows. Jackets are all shapes, from cropped to riding length; slacks are pleated and made out of drapable fabrics such as silk, flannel, lightweight wool, or crepe. When Murphy does wear a skirt, it's hemmed just above the knee, and accompanied by Donna Karan or Kenneth Cole flats. Off-hours, Calvin Klein jeans, vintage rayon shirts from the forties and fifties, turtlenecks from GAP, and flannel shirts from J. Crew are the rule. And in terms of jewelry, Stephen Dreck and Robert Lee Morris design most of Murphy's chunky bead necklaces. While Murphy tries to stay current, some trends will never be seen on her—for example, sheer tops over bras—thus ensuring that F.Y.I. stays easy on the I.

Q: Why does Murphy always wear something around her neck? Does she have age wrinkles on her throat? A scar from thyroid surgery? Or is it simply her "Teddy Kennedy at Mary Jo Kopechne's funeral" impression?

A: No on all three counts. Although Murphy may be pushing fifty, Hargate avows that she's not showing signs of age in her neck (where she *is* showing signs of age, he neglected to mention). "The reason we cover her neck," he explains, "is because she does a lot of screaming on the show—and when she gets excited, the veins pop out on her throat. It's better to cover them so the audience isn't distracted from what she's saying." Personally, we liked the Teddy Kennedy theory better.

Headliner: Bill McNeal (Phil Hartman)/*NewsRadio*.
Capsule summary: If he were a pie, he'd be rhubarb. If he were a

cake, he'd be layered. And if he were a cookie, he'd be damn lucky to have such a great job.

Body copy: Acerbic and chauvinistic, co-anchor Bill is a man of many layers. Clothes layers, that is. At the top of the multi-leveled list: vests. "He's got an attitude at the station," says LuEllyn Harper, the show's costumer. "The vests give him that extra air of seniority." He's also a monochromatic, tone-on-tone kind of guy in shades of brown and gray. To add dimension, Harper uses textured fabrics for his three-button suits (she fell in love with a Banana Republic three-piece suit that had cuffed, pleated trousers, and bought several of them) or sport jackets and trousers. Close to the vest, Bill's Donna Karan shirts are anything but white. "No one on the show wears white shirts," says Harper. "For Bill, I use muted plaids, or browns and grays with a subtle pattern." His ties, mostly Armani, have intricate prints, and are made of soft materials such as silk. "The main concept with Bill is mixing textures and patterns to give him a rich look," she says. "We have one sweater vest, but suit vests fit his personality better." Plus, they help us tell him apart from Frasier Crane.

Q: Why does Bill need to look so dapper when his audience can't see him? This is radio, for God's sake!

A: Because even radio announcers have to look good. This is television, for God's sake!

Headliner: Dave Nelson (Dave Foley)/*NewsRadio*.

Capsule summary: Kid from the midwestern hall hits the big city.

Body copy: The primary idea for Dave is "blue." Says Harper, "He's got blue eyes, and blue shirts look great on him, so I decided to make that his 'thing.'" She thinks it's a good color—a "powerful" color, even—for a young guy who's got a big station-director job. In addition to his "thing," he wears slightly conservative-yet-hip three-button suits from Hugo Boss,

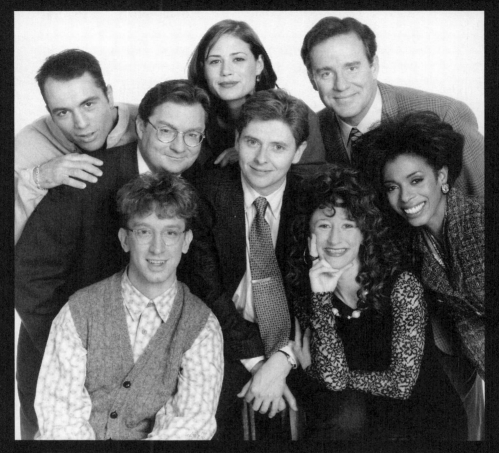

The *NewsRadio* gang signs on. Clockwise from the bespectacled nebbish at bottom left: Matthew (Andy Dick) gets vested; Joe (Joe Rogan) gears up for work; Jimmy James (Stephen Root) is a double-breasted man; Lisa (Maura Tierney) has a fit; Dave (Dave Foley) is tangled up in blue; Bill (Phil Hartman) is all plaid out; Catherine (Khandi Alexander) makes a perfect match; and Beth (Vicki Lewis) is sheer madness.

Photo: Courtesy of The National Broadcasting Company, Inc. Photographer: Chris Haston.

dress shoes, and strong ties. "There are so many guys in suits on the show, I have to distinguish them by their ties," says Harper. Dave's ties—usually by Calvin Klein, Donna Karan, and Nordstrom—are boldly hued and have geometric patterns such as, wait, don't tell us . . . squares?

Q: Does Dave ever really let his hair down?

A: Yes, but only when he's wearing a dress.

Headliner: Mike Flaherty (Michael J. Fox) / *Spin City*.

Capsule summary: Wee replica of a person is appointed deputy mayor.

Body copy: Although he has the weight of City Hall on his shoulders, Mike's suits have no discernible shoulder pads. That would be way too trendy for this politico. Much like his former alter ego, Alex P. Keaton, he favors traditional cuts and colors: navy and gray three-button suits, pleated trousers, dress shirts, and red power ties. Note that his tie is often slightly askew to reflect his harried-carried lifestyle, and his jackets are rarely buttoned. At home, he's the picture of casual in boxer shorts and T-shirts.

Q: What'll we do baby, without us? What'll we do baby, without us? 'Cause there ain't no nothing we can't love each other through—what'll we do baby, without us?

A: Sha la la la.

SPORTS PAGES

Headliner: Frank Fontana (Joe Regalbuto) / *Murphy Brown.*

Capsule summary: Danger Guy meets the Van Heusen Man.

Body copy: "Frank has the world's greatest collection of sport shirts," says Hargate, "many by Jhane Barnes and Calvin

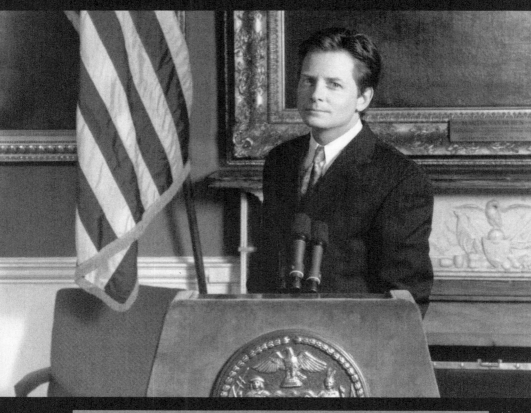

Michael J. Fox is a towering presence in *Spin City*, ABC's version of *The American President*, scaled down to small-screen proportions.

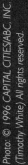

Klein." We're talking the entire range of shirts here, from dressy/dressy to dressy/casual to casual/dressy to casual/casual. It's mind-boggling/mind-boggling. Regardless of classification, they're all long-sleeved, made in soft fabrics, and tend to be dark (most of his ties are also on the dark side). Instead of suits, Frank goes for a blazer or sport coat with pleated slacks. When he's in casual/casual mode, chinos or jeans, flannel shirts by Joseph Abboud, and a bomber jacket are de rigueur. For footwear, Frank likes Bucks, Nike sneakers, and cowboy boots.

Q: What's a guy like that doing with so many shirts?

A: Wearing them. Why, what have you heard?

Headliner: Clark Kent/Superman (Dean Cain/Dean Cain)/*Lois and Clark.*

Capsule summary: By day, a mild-mannered reporter; by night, *buns of steel.*

Body copy: Clark's closet is about as ordinary as they come. "In the past, we've stuck with single-breasted, two-button sport coats by Hugo Boss and Canali," says Darryl Levine, the show's men's costume designer. "The jackets are dark hued, multi-colored, and usually textured." This season, Clark will get downright flashy (for him) in three- and four-button nubbly wool, crepe, and rayon suits, by Donna Karan, Hugo Boss, and Vestimenta. "I like his ties to be bright and loud," says Levine. "On television, you only see the top of the jacket and shirt—the tie should be bold enough to draw attention." When our hero's being casual, he lounges about in soft plaid shirts, jeans, T-shirts, and shorts. And when he's being super, he launches about in a stretch moleskin blue unitard (we mortals are more familiar with moleskin in the form of those small tan oval patches used to cover foot calluses, corns, blisters, etc.). His briefs are maroon moleskin

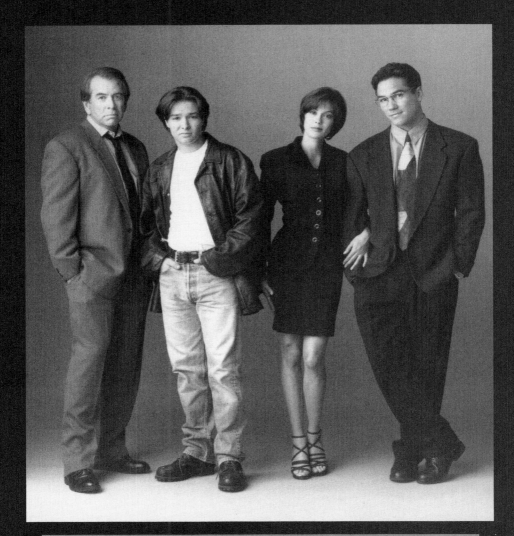

Journalism never looked so good. The four stars of *Lois and Clark* make the news, starting from the human column on the left: managing editor Perry White (Lane Smith) may not look happy, but photographer Jimmy Olsen (Justin Whalin) looks snappy; Lois (Teri Hatcher) looks strappy; and Clark (Dean Cain) looks, well, sappy. Happy?

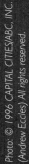

(it looks red on TV), and his cape is seven yards of light-weight wool in a slightly different shade of scarlet. The insignia on his chest is an enlarged version of the original, and his boots are custom-made of soft, hide leather with a hidden zipper down the back. "We go through about six to ten suits a year," says Levine. Naturally. All that changing in phone booths must wreak absolute havoc on your clothes.

Q: Uh, moleskin???

A: According to Levine, this soft, durable cotton fabric "dyes and fits well, and is a good, stretchy material. We don't have to add padding to the unitard at all—not in the shoulders, not in the thighs, not in the chest. And no, not in the trunks." Not that we were asking. Extra bonus: At the end of a long day of rescuing, when you peel that baby off—not a blister in sight!

HOME SECTION

Headliner: Corky Sherwood (Faith Ford) / *Murphy Brown*.

Capsule summary: Miss America goes to Washington.

Body copy: In the beginning, Corky was the quintessential dress-maker's mannequin in "tailored, fitted suits, right out of a beauty pageant," says Hargate. "I stopped short of putting her in gloves." Over time, however, she's matured into a more sophisticated character, and her clothes reflect this. "She's still got a younger look than Murphy, especially with the shorter hemlines," says Hargate. "I differentiate between the two women by putting Murphy in slacks, and casual separates." Corky's uniform usually consists of a suit or a pleated skirt and a blouse, over stockings or opaque tights. Her labels of choice include Ann Taylor, Bebe, and Adrienne

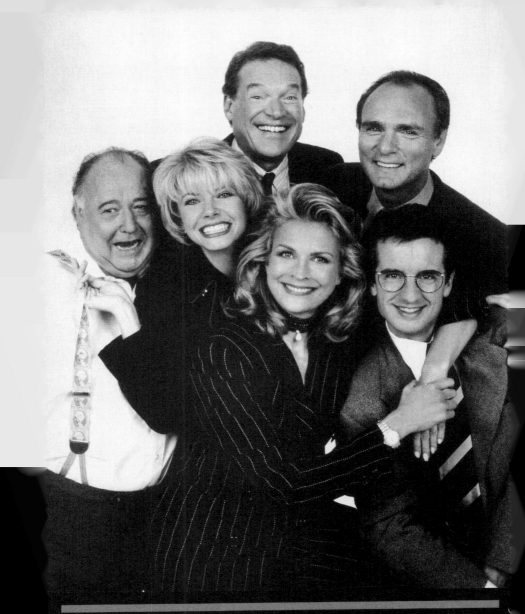

Look, ma, no cavities! The original FYI troop takes a bite out of prime time.
Clockwise from the now-defunct-so-we-won't-even-talk-about-him Miles on bottom right: Murphy (Candice Bergen) is a star in stripes; Corky (Faith Ford) is TV's
golden girl; Phil (Pat Corley) is defunct, too; Jim (Charles Kimbrough) is to Dial
for; and Frank (Joe Regalbuto) is waiting to pick up his shirts from the cleaners.

Vittadini. Also unlike Murphy, Corky does wear heels—most frequently, pumps with a little lift by Kenneth Cole.

Q: Does Corky ever wear pants?

A: "Maybe once, when they went on a field trip," says Hargate. "And I think she wore leggings and a sweater in the hurricane episode. But generally, we see her legs." Miles and Miles of them.

Headliner: Lisa Miller (Maura Tierney) / *NewsRadio.*

Capsule summary: MTM goes MTV.

Body copy: As a reporter, Lisa is supposed to be trendy, but sophisticated. Conservative, but with a twist. "Barneys is the best store for her," says Harper. She wears both zip-up straight-legged pants or wide-legged trousers, long and short skirts, and jackets of varying lengths. Current but timeless. Along with the Barneys store label, she has an Armani suit, and some Anne Klein and Calvin Klein separates, all in what Harper calls the medium tones: slate blue, moss green, brown, black, powder blue. Colorful, but subdued. She opts for stacked-heel loafers, dainty necklaces with single stone drops, and tiny stud earrings. "Whatever makes her seem professional but hip is fine," says Harper. "We alter every garment so the lines are clean. For one episode, I even took in a bulky pullover." Casual, but controlled.

Q: Is there anything about Lisa that doesn't involve a but?

A: Apparently not—unless you count Dave.

STYLE REPORT

Headliner: Lois Lane (Teri Hatcher) / *Lois and Clark.*

Capsule summary: It's a Dior, it's a Klein—it's Super Style!

Body copy: Yet another scholar of the classics, costume designer
Judith Curtis is "very conscious of choosing clothes that
won't seem dated in reruns. Right now, the tight, fitted look
is gone—this season, we're going easier." Donna Karan and
Christian LaCroix do their share, but Lois's main man of
the moment is Calvin Klein. "His clothes work on her," says
Curtis. "The long line of color—jacket and pants with
matching shoes and bag—makes her look taller." (Hatcher's
no peewee—she's five feet six—but her partner, Dean Cain,
is over six feet tall, so she needs the illusion of more
height.) Curtis's fondness for 1940s-style is evident in Lois's
suits with broad shoulders, wide lapels, and hemlines that
ride a few inches above the knee. "In the first season, we
made a lot of items reminiscent of that era," says Curtis. "We
still make a lot of her pants." Cigarette pants are the standard (you'll rarely find pleats on this girl reporter's size two
body), occasionally alternated with Banana Republic lightweight wool trousers. But it's on the color spectrum where
Lois really breaks out of the professional pack: "I don't do
much navy or black," says Curtis. "I like nut browns, but Teri
doesn't. We agree on dark red, muted sea foam green, pale
blue, muddy blue, and eggplant—I think it's called
aubergine these days." Stretch cotton, linen, and silk blouses
are in; harsh, itchy wool and corduroy are out. And
although the softness adds to Lois's sex appeal, "We don't
need to go overly low-cut or put her in sexy clothes," says
Curtis. "Let's face it, if she were wearing a giant sock, she'd
still be gorgeous." For formal occasions, Lois wears glamour
gowns from Badgley Mischka; on cold Gotham days she
wraps up with a cashmere trench coat. She'll track down a
lead in anything from high heels to Reeboks. And at home,
she opts for leggings, T-shirts, silk nighties, and flannel pj's,
depending on the season.

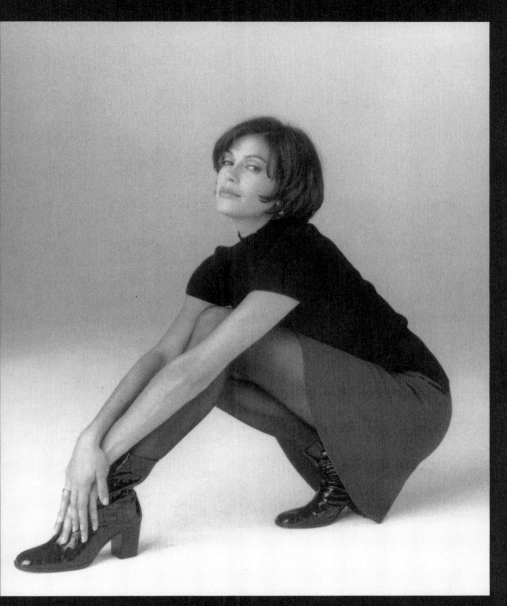

Lois and Clark's Teri Hatcher makes a long, lean headline in basic black. As always, she's the best-dressed woman on the planet. *The Daily Planet*, that is.

Q: When they're at home, since Clark has X-ray vision, why does she bother wearing clothes at all?

A: Because it may not be truth or justice, but it's the American way.

Headliner: Catherine Duke (Khandi Alexander) / *NewsRadio*.

Capsule summary: Giant hair on a stick.

Body copy: Not only a co-anchor, Catherine is a dedicated color coordinator. "Her shoes match her purse, her manicure matches her suit. Even her fake fur coats fit the scheme," says Harper. "She's that type of woman." Heels are high, skirts are short, and Ann Taylor, Emanuel Ungaro, DKNY, Christian Dior, Saks, and Neiman's provide her with showy suits. Lighter blues, yellows, pinks, creams, grays, and assorted animal prints spin her color wheel, and ample cleavage is a requirement. "It adds to her character," says Harper. "She has strong opinions and she's proud of her body."

Q: How is the average female supposed to react to a lithe, leggy dish like Khandi?

A: Oh, the usual way: denial, rage, despair, grief, hope, acceptance, and a fierce vow to start exercising right away. But first, a little TV.

WEATHER UPDATE

Headliner: Beth (Vicki Lewis) / *NewsRadio*.

Capsule summary: Another cockeyed, crazy caravan of a TV assistant.

Body copy: Convention be hanged; Beth is a fashion accident on purpose. "Anything I see that's wild and different says 'Beth' to me," explains Harper. "Her skirts are extremely short; she likes animal and reptile prints. Every week, I feel like I have to outdo last week's outfit. It can be stressful, but it's always

Be a *NewsRadio*-gram—or just look like one.

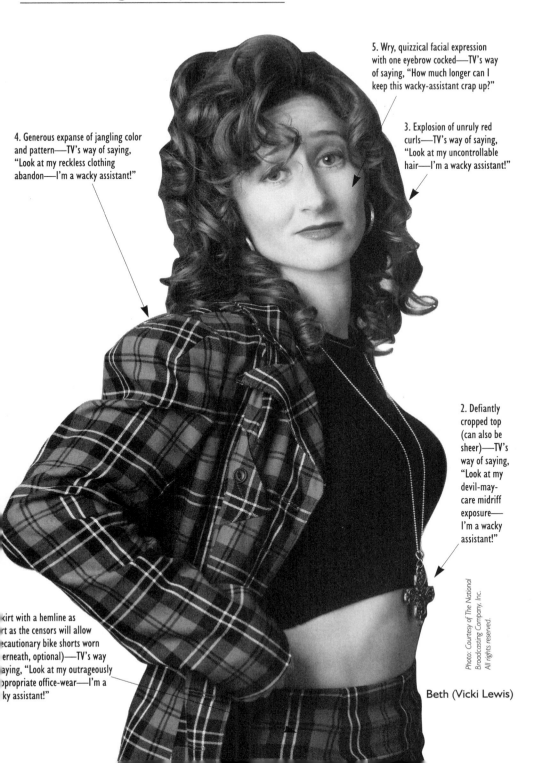

5. Wry, quizzical facial expression with one eyebrow cocked—TV's way of saying, "How much longer can I keep this wacky-assistant crap up?"

3. Explosion of unruly red curls—TV's way of saying, "Look at my uncontrollable hair—I'm a wacky assistant!"

4. Generous expanse of jangling color and pattern—TV's way of saying, "Look at my reckless clothing abandon—I'm a wacky assistant!"

2. Defiantly cropped top (can also be sheer)—TV's way of saying, "Look at my devil-may-care midriff exposure—I'm a wacky assistant!"

...irt with a hemline as ...rt as the censors will allow ...ecautionary bike shorts worn ...erneath, optional)—TV's way ...aying, "Look at my outrageously ...ppropriate office-wear—I'm a ...ky assistant!"

Beth (Vicki Lewis)

fun." Variety is the name of the game: a Gaultier top with a Dolce & Gabanna jacket, a Betsey Johnson skirt and Vivienne Tam top, an Anna Sui coat, a Diesel dress or a Bisou Bisou Mona Lisa silk-screened jacket. Stop the sensory stimulation, we think we're going to—mmph, bmph—puke. More downtown than upbeat, Beth wears plenty of black and shows scads of skin in bustiers, netting, and tight or cropped styles. Her taste in jewelry runs a silver streak via chain necklaces and hoop earrings. And she puts down her foot with zip-up ankle boots, lace-up boots or "a dressier version of combat boots." Whatever that means.

Q: Skirt-wise, how short will she go?

A: As short as the networks allow. "We measure the hems so they barely cover what they're meant to cover," says Harper. Lewis often wears cropped bike shorts underneath to protect against an accidental flash. Whether she's protecting herself or the viewers, we haven't decided.

Headliner: Matthew Brock (Andy Dick)/*NewsRadio.*

Capsule summary: Aesthetically challenged weirdo seeks refuge in the written word.

Body copy: Described by Harper as "an idiot savant of style," Matthew takes the vintage route in fifties and sixties sweaters and shirts, fuzzy pullovers, corduroys in autumn colors, and old plaid pants with suspenders. Because he occupies the broad comedy slot on the show, his clothes have to move. "He's the Chevy Chase of *NewsRadio,*" says Harper. "He does a lot of physical comedy and the clothes don't always survive his pratfalls. It's hard to get multiples of vintage clothes, so I get new stuff that looks old." Not your typical argyle-sweater geek, Matthew shops at Fred Segal, J. Crew, Banana Republic, and costume warehouses. The desired effect? "Funky and fun," says Harper.

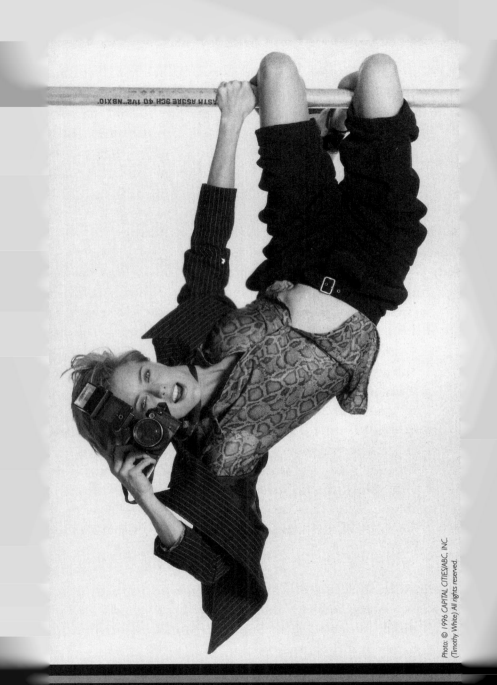

She oughtta be in pictures. *The Naked Truth*'s Tea Leoni is not-quite-naked enough as she changes clothes and careers at the speed of light. Click

Q: Does Matthew really have uncommonly big shoes, or is his over-all clownishness just playing tricks on our eyes?

A: An excellent question (if we do say so ourselves). "Andy has very wide feet," says Harper. "I tried to put him in Hush Puppies, but they were too painful, so he switched to two-tone Birkenstock shoes." Okay. And the reason for that haircut is . . . ?

Headliner: Nora Wilde (Tea Leoni) / *The Naked Truth.*

Capsule summary: Retro-Contempo-a-gogo. *So.*

Body copy: Poor-little-formerly-rich-girl Nora mixes pricey pieces from her past with thrift store purchases necessitated by her present financial strains. "But even when she was married to her millionaire, she liked kooky clothes," says costume design-er Louise Mingenbach. "The funky look is more expressive and artistic." Do tell. "She wears a lot of prints and weird com-binations. She'll mix a vintage suit with Isaac Mizrahi shoes, or a streamlined Calvin Klein suit with forties shoes." Mingenbach is inspired by two TV greats: Lucy and Mary. "Lucy wore exaggerated details—big shoulders, big pockets," she says, "Mary also wore extremes. That's what I try to do with Nora. I want her to look good and have energy."

Q: Exactly what kind of a name is Tea Leoni?

A: We couldn't really tell you, but all those vowels sure make it look cool.

Headliner: Susan Keane (Brooke Shields) / *Suddenly Susan.*

Capsule summary: Suddenly trendy. Suddenly slick. Suddenly sub-dued. Suddenly silly. Suddenly funky. Suddenly hip. Suddenly sorry you asked?

Body copy: When she left her lug of a boyfriend, Susan was sudden-ly single! When all the pilot scriptwriters got fired, her job as a book editor in San Diego suddenly became a job as a magazine columnist in San Francisco! And when her whole life changed, suddenly her clothes did, too! "Her style is going to evolve," says costume designer Bambi Breakstone of *Ellen* fame. "We started out with a debutante concept: Ralph Lauren jackets with brass buttons, white shirts, crepe trousers, Hush Puppies." Navy, brown, gray, turquoise, coral, aqua, black, and green are the colors to watch for, but don't get too attached to her Donna Karan cashmere sweaters, crepe double-breasted blazers, and scoop-necked sleeveless black dresses with pearls. "Every episode, she'll have a different style," promises Breakstone. In other words, she may go from black linen overalls to suddenly Armani! From TSE blouses to suddenly Dolce & Gabanna! With all this suddenness, she'd better have good treads on her shoes.

Q: What comes between Brooke and her Calvins?

A: Who gives a shit?

Oh, don't shake your finger at us. So, we made a little fun of Brooke Shields. Is this such a crime? What're you gonna do, arrest us for joking? Read us our Miranda rights? Lock us up and throw away the key? Tell us to stop, **In the Name of the Law**? Play along with us and turn to **Chapter 12**? Is that what you're gonna do? Is it? *Is it?*

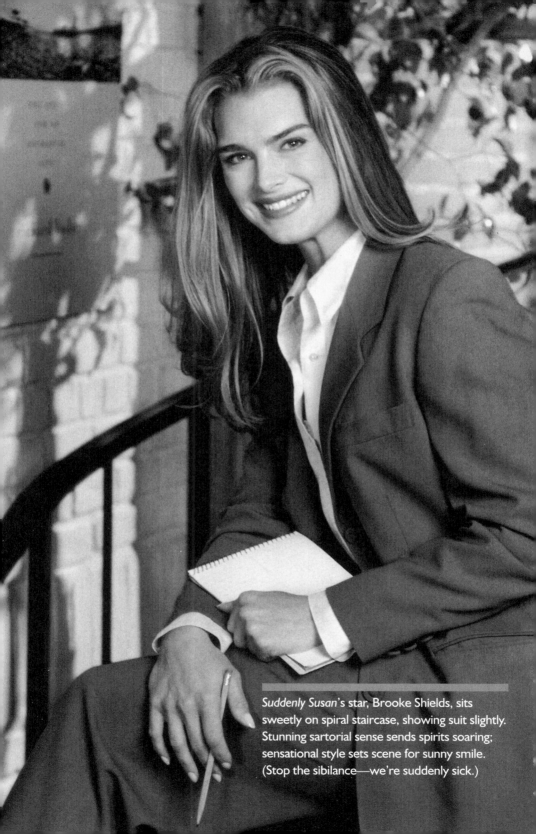

Suddenly Susan's star, Brooke Shields, sits
sweetly on spiral staircase, showing suit slightly.
Stunning sartorial sense sends spirits soaring;
sensational style sets scene for sunny smile.
(Stop the sibilance—we're suddenly sick.)

Chapter Twelve

In the Name of
the Law

WEDNESDAY, 10:00 P.M. (NBC) LAW & ORDER

(1990–present). Hour-long New York City–set drama in which a team
of detectives catches the bad guys, and a team of district attorneys
prosecutes them to the fullest extent of the script. First Amendment
finesse and work a day suits on display. Courtroom scenes a must-see.

TUESDAY, 10:00 P.M. (ABC) NYPD BLUE

(1993–present). Hour-long New York City–set drama in which a team
of detectives catches the bad guys, and sometimes gets caught with
their own pants down. Police vulgarity and short-sleeved shirts on display. Shower scenes a must-see.

SUNDAY, 9:00 P.M. (FOX) THE X-FILES

(1993–present). Hour-long variably set drama in which a team of FBI
agents catches aliens, vampires, mind pushers, psychics, thousand-year-
old shamans, as well as flack from their superiors. Conspiracy theories
and pant-suits on display. Abduction scenes a must-see.

[*Black screen. A faint red, white, and blue graphic appears at forefront of picture, and slowly draws back. Focus sharpens. Logo reads: NYPD Law & Made-to-Order Blue.*]

Voice-over: In the criminal fashion system, the people are represented by two separate yet equally important groups: the police, who wear clothes to investigate crime, and the district attorneys, who wear clothes to prosecute offenders. These are their stories.

[Ka-ching, ka-ching! *Sound of a cash register bell. Jump-cut to interior shot of Barneys New York. A crowd of people is milling around the counter, where a saleswoman sits, sobbing.*]

Saleswoman: . . . It all happened so fast—I was going over the day's receipts, when they walked up to me. The man pulled out a gun, and the woman pushed me into a dressing room. They forced me to, to (her voice quivers; she struggles to regain composure), to put on a beige linen suit with black wool tights and, and—oh, dear God, it's hard to even say it—white shoes! Then they made me tell one customer that it was okay to wear running shoes with a suit. And I had to persuade another woman to go to Chinatown and buy a fake Prada bag! *Fake Prada!* Ohmygodohmygod, I can't believe this happened! Why me, why now, why? (She bursts afresh into tears and pounds the register with her fists.)

[*The crowd parts as two men in black, three-button suits stride purposefully up the aisle.*]

Bystander (whispering excitedly): It's the fashion police!
Saleswoman (suddenly frosty): This cash register is closed, gentlemen—you'll have to make your purchases elsewhe—
First officer (interrupting): You can save your attitude for the paying customers, Ma'am. (Flashes his badge.) So, the couple

that approached you—what did they look like? Short guy with a mustache? Tall, thin woman with skunked hair?

Saleswoman: Yes, yes, exactly! Do you know them?

First Officer (exchanging meaningful glance with partner): Yeah, we know 'em.

Second Officer (nodding): We know 'em, all right. Sounds like T. J. Maxx and Annie Sez are out on the streets again.

[*Quick fade and cut back to black screen with logo. Synthesizer theme music kicks in. Camera pans along New York City skyline. Series of gritty black-and-white photographs of characters slowly flashes on screen—first the police officers, then the lawyers. Images are clothes-captioned for the style-impaired. Credits roll.*]

THE COPS

[*Wide opening shot of Manhattan's One Police Plaza. Rhythmic bass line picks up.*]

Image of: Detective Bobby Simone/*NYPD Blue.* He is long, lean, and smoldering in an elegant Italian suit.

Large type reads: JIMMY SMITS.

Caption reads: Overall effect is slick yet classic. Character wears designer suits from Hugo Boss and Donna Karan. Shirts by Calvin Klein, Armani, and Barneys store brand are often textured to add dimension. Garments are never made of hard-pressed fabric; instead, textured materials such as wool crepe, linen crepe, and twill are used. Pants always have a reverse box pleat; jackets are always single-breasted with two buttons.

Color panel: Palette is "controlled"—olive, brown, taupe and gray.

Be an *NYPD Blue*-print—or just look like one.

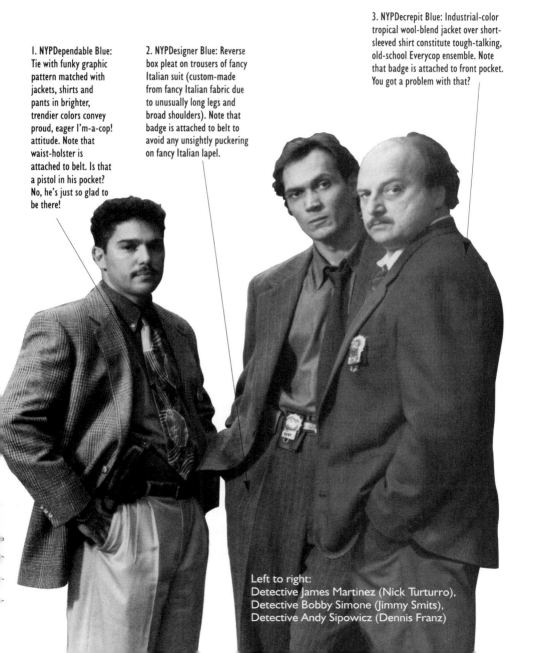

3. NYPDecrepit Blue: Industrial-color tropical wool-blend jacket over short-sleeved shirt constitute tough-talking, old-school Everycop ensemble. Note that badge is attached to front pocket. You got a problem with that?

1. NYPDependable Blue: Tie with funky graphic pattern matched with jackets, shirts and pants in brighter, trendier colors convey proud, eager I'm-a-cop! attitude. Note that waist-holster is attached to belt. Is that a pistol in his pocket? No, he's just so glad to be there!

2. NYPDesigner Blue: Reverse box pleat on trousers of fancy Italian suit (custom-made from fancy Italian fabric due to unusually long legs and broad shoulders). Note that badge is attached to belt to avoid any unsightly puckering on fancy Italian lapel.

Left to right:
Detective James Martinez (Nick Turturro),
Detective Bobby Simone (Jimmy Smits),
Detective Andy Sipowicz (Dennis Franz)

Technical notes: According to costume designer Brad Loman, "Smits has extra-broad shoulders and long limbs—nothing off the rack fits him. My tailor has to take the clothes apart and put them back together again." Sometimes, Loman buys the fabric directly from the manufacturers—for example, he purchased a length of Armani crepe fabric and made several pairs of pants with it. In addition, Smits has size-thirteen feet.

Final take: You know what they say about men on TV with big feet, don't you? Big Rock . . . ports.

Image of: Detective Andy Sipowicz/*NYPD Blue.* He is the quintessential old-school, tough-talking cop with a heart of gold—a big teddy bear with a big, big gun.

Large type reads: DENNIS FRANZ.

Caption reads: Sipowicz should represent Everycop. "He always wears bad suits," says Loman. "I shop for him at Sears or Moe Ginsburg." Jackets are square cut and single-breasted, in tropical wool blends; they're combined with flat-front pants, striped ties, and Rockports.

Color panel: Mousy blues, dirty browns, and other industrial shades.

Technical notes: Even in the dead of winter, short-sleeved shirts are the rule. "We cut the sleeves of regular dress shirts so we have more to choose from," says Loman.

Final take: Cold arms, warm heart.

Image of: Detective Diane Russell/*NYPD Blue.* She is attractive, but not excessively chic.

Large type reads: KIM DELANEY.

Caption reads: Character leans heavily on a design line from Nordstrom called Greta Garbo—and on her, Garbo talks. Pant suits are the favored apparel, with dark sweaters and blouses. Footwear consists primarily of Charles David and

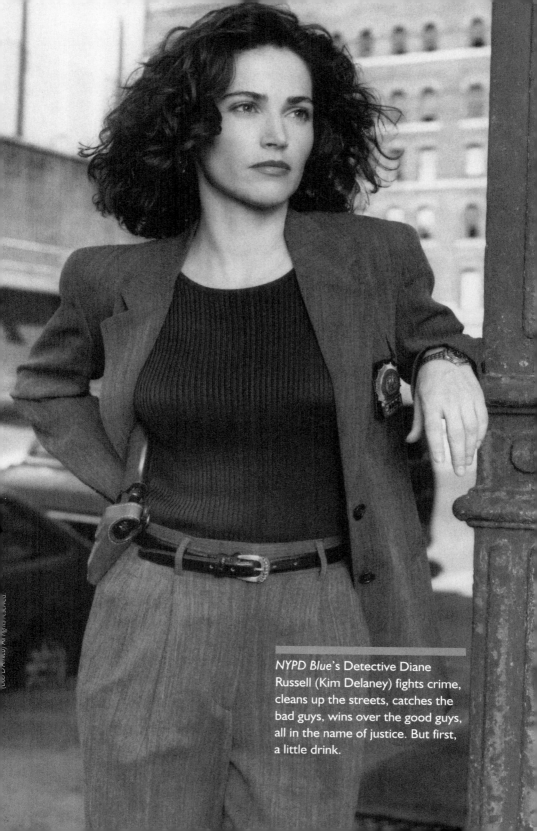

NYPD Blue's Detective Diane Russell (Kim Delaney) fights crime, cleans up the streets, catches the bad guys, wins over the good guys, all in the name of justice. But first, a little drink.

DKNY loafers.

Color panel: Earth tones.

Technical notes: Although Delaney is a diminutive size two, she has no clothes that are extremely fitted. Jackets must accommodate waist holster; trousers are fitted through the hip with a bit of fullness in the leg. "The legs can't have too much extra fabric, though," says Loman. "We don't want to see her pants flapping in the wind when she chases after a criminal."

Final take: Stop, in the name of the—flapflapflap—law!

Image of: Detective Lennie Briscoe/*Law & Order*. His clothes are slightly outdated and weathered—as is he.

Large type reads: JERRY ORBACH.

Caption reads: Briscoe is the kind of guy who goes to Yonkers Raceway on his day off. Consequently, costume designer Jennifer von Mayrhaufer originated his wardrobe in Stern's department store in Yonkers. Currently, she also shops at Moe Ginsburg and Saks for Briscoe's two-button, single-breasted sport jackets, straight, unpleated pants, and long- and short-sleeved shirts.

Color panel: Understated blues, greens, beiges, and browns.

Technical notes: Belt matches shoes; ties are in the same solid color as jackets. No fashion developments are anticipated: "His sense of style was set a few decades ago," says von Mayrhaufer, "and it's not going to change." Nonetheless, viewers should not be fooled by humdrum appearance; Orbach is literally a sharpshooter. For last season's finale, the actor bragged so much about his billiards prowess, producers had a pool-table scene written in—and Orbach performed right on cue.

Final take: Is that an eight ball in your corner pocket, or are you just glad to see us?

Image of: Detective Reynaldo Curtis/*Law & Order.* He is long, lean, and smouldering—the NBC man's Jimmy Smits.

Large type reads: BENJAMIN BRATT.

Caption reads: Curtis walks his beat in style. "For a detective, his clothes are hip-looking," says von Mayrhaufer. He prefers suits to sport jackets, and he likes designers over department store brands. Hugo Boss, in particular, fits the bill for sharp, elegant single-breasted suits. For textured two- or three-button jackets, as well as ties, Curtis leans toward Italian designers such as Armani.

Color panel: Dark—gray, black, navy, and dark green.

Technical notes: Shirts should be of the highest quality—they may be striped or solid, but never have button-down collars. Script writers, please note that character can afford to indulge his expensive tastes because he married a woman of considerable means.

Final take: You can beat an egg, you can beat a drum—but you can't beat a wife with a lot of money.

Image of: Lieutenant Anita Van Buren/*Law & Order.* She is conservative and quietly imposing.

Large type reads: S. EPATHA MERKERSON.

Caption reads: As a black female boss to a bunch of white men, Van Buren holds her ground in traditional garb. "We see her as the kind of woman who goes to big department stores like Macy's and buys clothes in bulk," says von Mayrhaufer. While skirts and blouses are standard issue, she occasionally wears pants in silk or rayon with her usual dignified pumps.

Color panel: Subdued earth tones.

Technical notes: Skirts are strictly knee-length; pants and blouses are never tight. Character strives for effect, not affect. For further grounding in reality, over a dozen real-life police officers have played various members of Van Buren's precinct on the show.

Final take: So, where was she when New York's Finest were trashing the Washington Hyatt Regency?

THE LAWYERS

[*Cut to exterior shot of City Hall. Synthesized wind instrument weaves soulful yet contemplative melody.*]

Image of: Assistant District Attorney Sylvia Costas/*NYPD Blue.* Sleekly outfitted, she looks polished and professional.

Large type reads: SHARON LAWRENCE.

Caption reads: Most of Costas's suits are custom-made, in a cut that Loman refers to as "business classic." She will show her legs in short skirts; jackets are single- and double-breasted, with blouses underneath. Jewelry is discreet, shoes are moderately heeled pumps.

Color panel: Butter yellow, amber, rust, and gray, supplemented with emerald or blue.

Technical notes: Blouses and jackets are stalwartly buttoned up. A professional air should be maintained at all times, especially since the character is married to Detective Sipowicz and any appearance of favoritism must be avoided.

Final take: If she's married to him, why in God's name doesn't she do something about those short-sleeved shirts?

Image of: Assistant District Attorney Jack McCoy/*Law & Order.* He is unassuming, but wily as a very disheveled fox.

Large type reads: SAM WATERSTON.

Caption reads: Day-to-day, McCoy goes for tweed single-breasted

Be a *Law & Orderly*—or just look like one.

1. Lost in Paradise: Fashion perfection in the form of three-button Italian suit, dress shirt, and Armani tie. Stop, in the name of the Polizia!

4. Lost in Thought: Fashion apathy in the form of terminally wrinkled shirt and generic Brooks Brothers–ish sack suit.

2. Lost in Yonkers: Fashion throwback in the form of outmoded two-button sport coat and nondescript tie. Not seen in breast pocket: OTB racing form.

3. Lost.

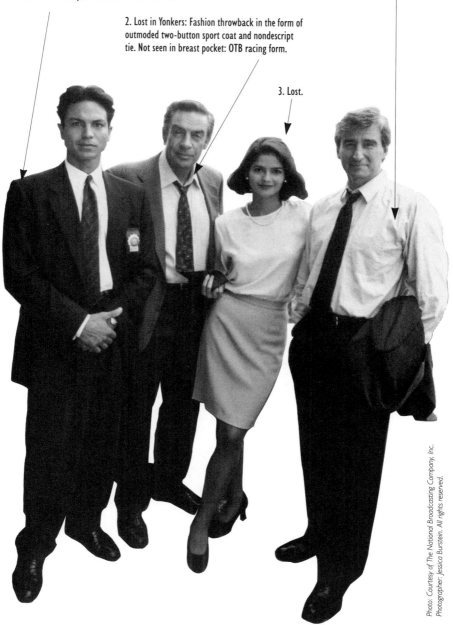

Left to right: Detective Reynaldo Curtis (Benjamin Bratt), Detective Lennie Briscoe (Jerry Orbach), Assistant D.A. Claire Kinkaid (Jill Hennessy), Assistant D.A. Jack McCoy (Sam Waterston)

jackets and striped shirts. In court, he'll wear a more expensive two-button single-breasted suit (he owns two—one blue, one gray), with a light shirt and a Brooks Brothers club tie.

Color panel: Neutral—cream, taupe, gray, slate blue.

Technical notes: Character should be terminally rumpled. According to von Mayrhaufer, "He sees his work clothes as a uniform that he has to wear, but doesn't have to maintain well."

Final take: Little hint? Permanent press.

Image of: Assistant District Attorney Jamie Ross/*Law & Order.* The new kid on the block, she has taken the office by sartorial storm.

Large type reads: CAREY LOWELL.

Caption reads: Ross is the only DA who dresses expensively, mainly in Calvin Klein. In court, she wears black suits; in the office, she wears black sweaters, skirts, and trousers. She paces the courtroom in DKNY heeled loafers, and walks through City Hall in Isaac Mizrahi flats.

Color panel: Black.

Technical notes: The concept behind Ross's closet is that she was once a legal shark who was married to a high-powered corporate lawyer. Although she is now simplifying her life as an assistant DA, her clothes are still a reflection of paychecks past.

Final take: Easy on the eye—but she ain't no Jill Hennessy.

Image of: District Attorney Adam Schiff/*Law & Order.* He is cynical and aesthetically unextraordinary.

Large type reads: STEVEN HILL.

Caption reads: Schiff's wardrobe is plain and conventional: a shifting collection of simple dress shirts and English suits.

Color panel: Refined neutrals.

Technical notes: All clothes must be approved by a rabbi before they are worn. This is not a joke: In real life, actor Steven Hill is an Orthodox Jew, and adheres to the laws of his religion. One of these laws decrees that you cannot mix linen and wool—unfortunately, many wool suits have a linen interface. So, von Mayrhaufer keeps a rabbi on call to check Hill's wardrobe for *shatnes* standards (the clothing equivalent of kosher). If the garments measure up, the rabbi will then sew a label inside it that reads, "*Shatnes*-approved by Rabbi Hollywood [not his real name]."

Final take: Quick fact for TV buffs: Hill was the original leader of the *Mission: Impossible* crew, but was fired after one season for refusing to work on the Sabbath, and replaced by Peter Graves. Apparently, God isn't an Equity member.

[*Action shot of entire group walking together. Sipowicz and Briscoe are comparing short-sleeved shirt prices. Curtis and Ross are discussing the shopping benefits of having a wealthy spouse. Van Buren and Costas are trying on each other's pumps. Schiff smiles benignly—he answers to a higher order. Theme song winds down. Fade to black. Prepare for opening sequence of next show.*]

Standard-length commercial break: Jeep Cherokee, Dr. Pepper, Excedrin, Bounty Paper Towels, Excedrin again, American Express, McDonald's, Pepcid AC, teaser for the local news, Lexus, Revlon, Coors Light.

[*Immediate flash to first scene. Evening. Exterior shot of strip mall. Chiron scrolls out at bottom of the screen: Fat City, just outside Burbank, California. Move to interior shot. We see a large room filled with racks of oversized clothing; a signed photograph of Roseanne is taped behind the cash register. A young, male salesclerk is closing up for the night. As he turns off the lights, he notices a large, glowing sphere in the millinery department.*]

Salesclerk: What the—?

[*Puzzled, he approaches it. The sphere becomes brighter, more defined—it almost resembles a giant head. Hat-stands begin to shake; one by one, hats float up to the top of the head, and then appear to be flung through the air by some unseen force. There is a flash of green fire and a puff of smoke.*]

Salesclerk: AAAGGGHHH! (He blacks out.)

[*Black screen with full-bleed gray-and-white logo. Logo reads: The X-LARGE Files. Photo sequence: Grainy, freeze-frame images of flying caftan—writhing waistband—screaming woman trying on bathing suit—headline reading Paranormal Apparel—suit without a body floating up stairway—headline reading Lagerfeld Denies Knowledge—outline of mannequin—close-up of collar button—bolt of lightning—slow-motion shot of credit card falling into hand—slogan: The Girth Is Out There. Credits roll.*]

Image of: Agent Fox Mulder/*The X-Files*. He is a slight man with a penetrating gaze.

Large type reads: DAVID DUCHOVNY.

Caption reads: To compensate for the lack of color in Mulder's wardrobe (see Color panel, below), costume designer Jenni Gullett strives for texture and a compelling silhouette. "He wears primarily lightweight-wool Hugo Boss suits, dress shirts, and pleated trousers," she says, "with muted print ties—mostly Armani." Mulder has a collection of Armani and Boss overcoats, as well as a few leather car coats, and an Eddie Bauer winter jacket. Off-hours, he likes V-neck cashmere sweaters, mock turtlenecks, Levi's 501s, J. Crew T-shirts, and other filler items from GAP. And on his globetrotting feet, he sticks to orthopedically correct shoes from Ecco, or sneakers.

Color panel: "Gloomy neutrals"—gray, dark blue, and black, with a

Be an X-phile—or just look like one.

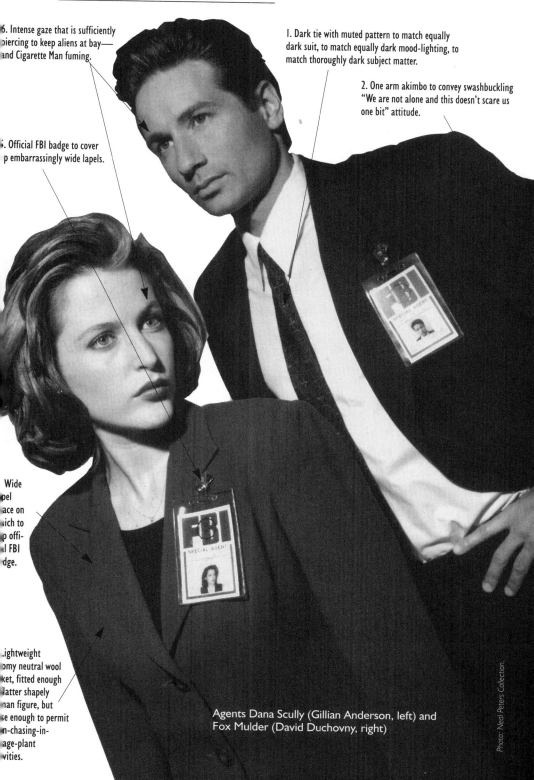

6. Intense gaze that is sufficiently piercing to keep aliens at bay—and Cigarette Man fuming.

1. Dark tie with muted pattern to match equally dark suit, to match equally dark mood-lighting, to match thoroughly dark subject matter.

2. One arm akimbo to convey swashbuckling "We are not alone and this doesn't scare us one bit" attitude.

5. Official FBI badge to cover up embarrassingly wide lapels.

Wide lapel space on which to top official FBI badge.

Lightweight roomy neutral wool jacket, fitted enough to flatter shapely human figure, but loose enough to permit alien-chasing-in-foliage-plant activities.

Agents Dana Scully (Gillian Anderson, left) and Fox Mulder (David Duchovny, right) few shirts in white and light blue. "The show has a unique style of lighting," says Gullett. "The dark lighting and blue glow have created a new look for TV, which is good. But all the details of the clothes are subsequently lost, which is bad."

Technical notes: Clothing is consistently baggy; character's suits are imprecisely fitted such that they appear to be a size too big. "Of course, we could get his suits tailored," says Gullet, "but Mulder would never waste time like that. He'd buy and fly." Furthermore, supplies of ooze, blood, dirt, and other viscous substances should be kept on hand to splatter on garments. For instance, when Mulder kneels on the ground to examine an unearthed grave, trousers should be suitably soiled for next scene. Note: Mulder kneels on only his right knee.

Final take: Meanwhile, when was the last time you read instructions that said "trousers should be *suitably soiled?*"

Image of: Agent Dana Scully/*The X-Files.* She is a slight woman with a penetrating gaze.

Large type reads: GILLIAN ANDERSON.

Caption reads: Scully is more conservative than her partner, intellectually and sartorially. She favors pant suits, especially for scenes where she'll be called on to do stunts such as running around in a sewage plant chasing pod creatures. "The better part of her closet consists of suits by two local [Vancouver] designers: Feizal Virani and Jacqueline Conior," says Gullett. Her skirts are knee length—standard FBI requirements; her trousers are narrow but not straight all the way down (again, the sewage plant/pod-creature influence). Scully has been a fan of duster coats, but recently, she's switched to a Banana Republic knee-length fitted coat. Her casual garb is equally conservative: tapered, pleated dress pants or DKNY jeans, a cardigan, and a ribbed crew-neck T-shirt from GAP. Police-sanctioned pumps or J. Crew lace-up ankle boots are her preferred footnotes.

Color panel: More gloomy neutrals—earth tones, black, navy, and green. Even so, she always appears brighter than Mulder because of her red hair, bright blue eyes, and pale skin.

Technical notes: Lightweight wool jackets are meticulously fitted to make character seem taller (Anderson is only five feet two). "When we get her pieces in, we do a huge number of alterations—she's the opposite of Mulder in that way," says Gullett. Small round glasses should be worn when character is using FBI computers, and Lucite protective eyewear is required for autopsies. Signature jewelry is a tiny gold cross—the same gold cross that Mulder kept as a memento during the episodes when Scully was dead.

Final take: Of course, everyone knew she wasn't *really* dead—she was just pregnant in real life, and written off the show until she had her baby.

[*Jump cut to second scene. Interior shot of Fat City millinery department, two days later. Agents Mulder and Scully are interviewing the salesclerk.*]

Mulder: So, did the head threaten you, or harm you in any way?

Salesperson: No, it was benign.

Mulder: And you passed out because . . . ?

Salesperson: Because I was scared, okay? Look, I'm just a regular guy—I'm not some FBI maniac who's thrilled at the idea of a giant head.

Mulder: Actually, I'm thrilled at the idea of a little head.

Scully (examining a hat-stand)**:** Mulder, over here. (Mulder walks over to where Scully is standing.) I see traces of a transparent, oily substance with white flakes. I'm not sure what it is—I'll have to identify it at the lab.

Mulder: You know damn well what it is, Scully. It's the same substance we found at Lard Bodies, and Crisco Kids, and that store in Cleveland—Buy Stuff Here, You Massive Load of Excess Flesh. The salespeople there all had the exact same encounter with a giant head. Why can't you accept that we have either a roving protoplasmic specter or a migrant extraterrestrial on our hands?

Scully: I admit there's a correlation, but I need proof. Scientific proof.

Salesperson (perking up): Did someone say Cleveland? When I was cleaning up today, I found this. (He hands Mulder a piece of paper. It is covered with diagrams and numbered questions—a college physics exam from a university in Ohio. Written at the top of the exam: Physics 101. Professor Dick Soloman. Mulder hands the paper to Scully.) Right before I closed up that night, a guy was milling around near the hats. He must have dropped this before he left.

Mulder: Can you give us a description?

Salesperson: Well, he looked a lot like John Lithgow.

Scully (exchanging a meaningful glance with Mulder): Thank you, Mr. Salesperson. We'll be in touch. (They exit the store.)

Mulder: Is that proof enough for you? Or are you going to tell me that John Lithgow look-alikes are shopping for caftans all over the country?

Scully (punching numbers into her cell phone): Sergeant Skinner? Agent Mulder and I are going to Cleveland. We have reason to believe that, as inhabitants of the third rock from the sun, we are not alone. (She hangs up, turns to Mulder, and sighs.) When's the next flight to Ohio? Book us in coach— if I put anything else on my credit card, I'll have to declare **Chapter 13**.

Mulder: Eleven. Bankruptcy is chapter eleven.

Scully: Whatever. Either way, the airfare's going to be **Out of This World**.

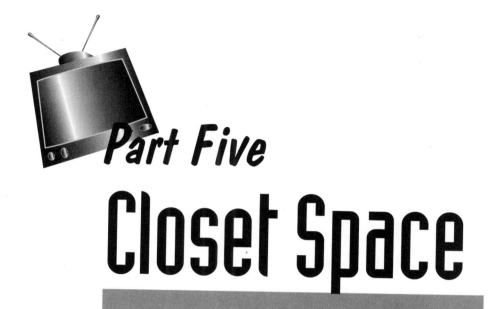

Part Five
Closet Space

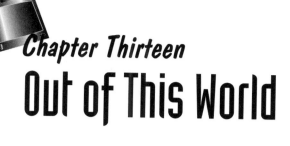

Chapter Thirteen
Out of This World

SATURDAY, 9:00 P.M. (SYNDICATED) XENA: WARRIOR PRINCESS

(1995–present). Ancient Greek Amazon kicks evil-doing butt all over the Aegean. Dominatrix fashion, lots of leather, and a bad attitude.

SATURDAY, 8:00 P.M. (SYNDICATED) HERCULES: THE LEGENDARY JOURNEYS

(1994–present). Ancient Greek quarterback kicks immortal evil-doing butt, all over Olympus. Rugged fashion, more leather, and a bad haircut.

SATURDAY, 7:00 P.M. (SYNDICATED) STAR TREK: DEEP SPACE NINE

(1993–present). Intergalactic peacekeeping force kicks war-mongering Kardasian butt all over space station. Uniform fashions, ear jewelry, and a bad time slot.

WEDNESDAY, 9:00 P.M. (UPN) STAR TREK: VOYAGER

(1995–present). Lost-in-space starship kicks itself because it can't figure out how to get back home to Earth. Jumpsuit fashions, sleek buns, and a bad sense of direction.

SUNDAY, 8:00 P.M. (NBC) THIRD ROCK FROM THE SUN

(1996–present). Four aliens in a strange land kick around in Ohio college town. Salvation Army fashions, comic aesthetic, and a bad blow for ABC.

niforms used to be a big deal on television. The cops on *Adam-12* wore uniforms. *Hogan's Heroes* wore uniforms. *CHiPs, Gomer Pyle,* the doctors on *M*A*S*H,* the *Love Boat* crew, even the waitresses at Mel's Diner wore uniforms. Nowadays, uniforms have been replaced by . . . multiforms. Cops wear everything from Armani to Zegna. Doctors choose from a rainbow of scrubs. Waitresses sport fabulous haircuts and might throw on a cute apron if it happens to look good with their outfit. As for military personnel, they got shipped out to Made-for-TV-Movieland years ago. If you're craving a glimpse of uniform, you've got only two areas of recourse: sports and space.

Which makes sense, if you think about it. In both sports and space teams, the members are working toward a common goal. Each member has a specific position or post, you get flurries of activity with breaks in between, strategy involves equal parts offense and defense, and there's always a captain. Sports requires space, space requires sport (okay, maybe they call them *ports,* but it's the exact same thing, just with the *S* moved around). Plus, a lot of the people are constantly trying to figure out how to get home. You might recall that one of the big science fiction movies of our time was actually titled *Star Trek IV: The Voyage Home.* Obvious title choice for the next installment? *Star Trek V: Unpacking.* Not that anyone listened to us (they ended up calling it—huge eye roll—*The Final Frontier*), but it does bring us quite nicely to our own final frontier: out-of-this-world fashion.

The fact is, whether you're a space voyager, an ancient Greek superhero, or simply a displaced alien trying to eke out an honest

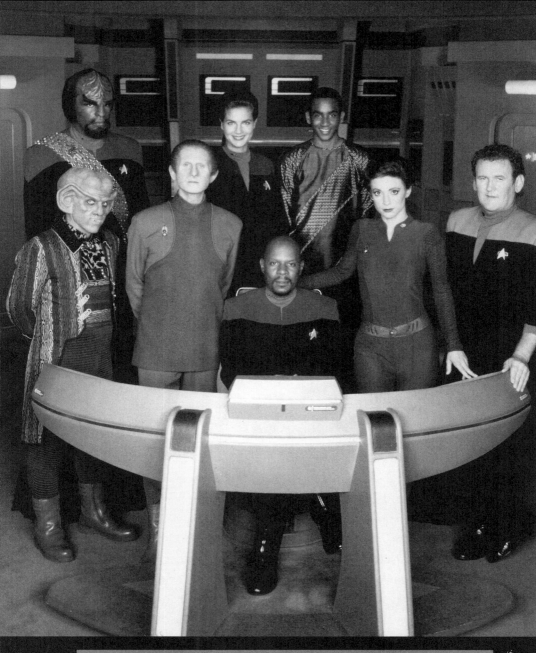

Eight is enough on *Star Trek: Deep Space Nine*. Now that they're all suited up—bridge, anyone?

living as a college professor, you've got to wear clothes if you want to be on TV. For starters, it's the law. Plus, if you cavorted around naked, people might catch on to the fact that you're really some mere mortal actor masquerading as a Bajoran or a Borg (or possibly even a Björn Borg). Here, a guide to some of the most popular otherworldly characters and their team uniforms. Remember: you're not just in the major league now—you're in the Ursa Major league.

The Federation Team

Team captains: Captain Benjamin Sisko (Avery Brooks)/*Star Trek: Deep Space Nine*; Captain Kathryn Janeway (Kate Mulgrew)/*Star Trek: Voyager.*

Roster: All deep-space voyagers who are operatives for the peace-seeking United Intergalactic Federation of Planets. From the *DS9* rotation: Medical Officer Dr. Julian Bashir (Alexander Siddig), Lieutenant Commander Worf (Michael Dorn), Science Officer Jadzia Dax (Terry Farrell), Chief Operations Officer Miles O'Brien (Colm Meaney). From the *Voyager* rotation: First Officer Chakotay (Robert Bletran), Tactical/Security Officer Tuvok (Tim Russ), Chief Engineer B'Elanna Torres (Roxann Biggs-Dawson), Lieutenant Junior Grade Tom Paris (Robert Duncan McNeill) and Op/Communications Officer Harry Kim (Garrett Wang).

Uniform: According to longtime costume designer Robert Blackman, the standard-issue Federation uniform consists of a long-sleeved black jumpsuit of lightweight wool gabardine. An elastic casing on the sides allows the actors greater movement. The jumpsuit is fit from the ankle to the jewel-neckline; the front panel can be unzipped a few inches on top. "Everyone wears some degree of shoulder pad," says Blackman. "How much depends on the individual actor's form." Underneath, the actors wear gray mock turtlenecks.

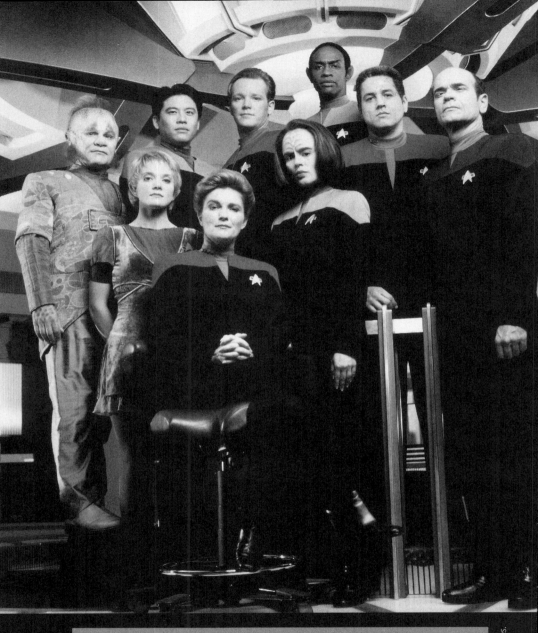

The fairly uniform cast of *Star Trek: Voyager*, led by Captain Janeway (Kate Mulgrew, front center). They said they were just going around the corner for a cup of coffee—and never came back!

Blackman's closet inspiration? NASA. "We envisioned that the clothing of the future would be sleek and offer comfort and mobility," says Blackman. "For us, though, it's more the illusion of comfort—wool gabardine can be incredibly hot, and I imagine it gets pretty uncomfortable after a twelve-hour shoot."

The color bars—the strip of color that runs horizontally across the jumpsuit's shoulders—correspond with the character's assignment. A red color bar (it's actually maroon, but looks red on TV) indicates that the character holds a command post—e.g., Sisko, Janeway, Worf, and Chakotay. A blue color bar (really teal) denotes a medical or scientific post—e.g., Dax and Bashir. A gold color bar (really yellowish) means the character is in engineering or security—e.g., O'Brien, Torres, Tuvok, Kim. For all we know, the bars themselves are actually big round circles that just look like bars. *That's the magic of television.*

On the right side of each character's turtleneck, a combination of gold and black dots (on *Voyager*, they're closer to dashes) signifies his or her rank. The ranking system: Captains wear four gold dots; commanders wear three gold dots; lieutenant commanders wear two gold dots and one black dot. Two gold dots mean lieutenant; one gold and one black dot mean lieutenant junior grade, one gold dot means ensign. Four raised dots mean the letter G. Three dots, three dashes, and three dots mean S.O.S. Many tiny red dots mean chicken pox. And so on. At the bottom of the totem pole, chief petty officers, sergeants, and enlisted men make do with small patches; none of the Federation members wears any jewelry—not even wedding rings.

Spoilers: The Bajoran and the Ferengi. The deeply religious Bajorans focus most of their energy on keeping the evil, totalitarian Kardasians from inhabiting their planet. And although the *DS9* Federation helps them in their battle, the

Bajorans are still suspicious of the seemingly secular Federation commanders. (Yeah, our brains are spinning, too.) First Officer Kira Nerys (Nana Visitor), the second-in-command at *DS9*'s space station and former freedom fighter/terrorist against the Kardasians, acts as a bridge between the two peoples. Her uniform—standard Bajoran military garb—consists of a one-piece rust-and-gray spandex jumpsuit with epaulet sleeves (the epaulets are so exaggerated, they resemble a hunting yolk). She even has special alien lingerie. "The spandex is stretched so tight, we had to custom-design a bra for her," says Blackman. "It's made of foam, and has a high cut with no seams." Kira also wears the traditional Bajoran bauble—an ear cuff with a chain that dangles and connects to her clip-on earring. Her colleague, Security Officer Odo (René Auberjonois), the shape-shifting space-station constable, dresses more civilian in a brown-and-tan jacket-and-pants ensemble. On his feet, he sticks to bucket boots. Apparently, Rockports haven't made it out to Bajor.

The big-skulled, big-eared capitalist Ferengi don't work against the Federation—they work to exploit it. Quark (Armin Shimerman), who runs the gaming operation on DS9's space station, "dresses in the romantic period, with saturated-color high-collared jackets cut short at the waist," says Blackman. Little brocade vests and frilly shirts complete the picture. "I think of the Ferengi as being well-dressed ferrets," says Blackman. "Ferrets that are dandified in a twenty-fourth-century kind of way." *Quelle* romance.

League Standing: With millions of Trekkies across the world, the Federation team will most likely continue to score high, provided there's still undiscovered country to explore. Or, provided we can hold on to enough brain cells to figure out what the hell they're talking about.

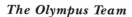

The Olympus Team

Team captains: Xena (Lucy Lawless) and Hercules (Kevin Sorbo).

Roster: Gabrielle (Renee O'Connor) and Iolaus (Michael Hurst).

Uniform: Front and center, female team captain Xena wears a studded leather-and-gold backless breastplate. Evidently, it provides her with support of mythic proportions—no matter how emphatically she's trampling the bad guys, you'll never see her jiggle. Her miniskirt is made of leather straps adorned with matching studs; accessories include black leather boots with knee guards, leather upper-arm bands, and black leather-and-silver wrist guards. She also carries a whip, a sword, and a hollow tempered-steel Frisbee doohickey that she flings with incredible accuracy. Sidekick Gabrielle, the storyteller, is more of a Contempo Colosseum kind of girl. She wears a low-slung suede miniskirt, a short-sleeved suede midriff-baring tunic, and woven boots with laces that wind around the ankle and calf. Since she isn't overly fond of accessories, she prefers not to carry any implements of torture.

Hercules, the male captain, is also way into cow-hide (memo to all you cows out there: Hide!). His brown leather pants are dominated by woven chaps—to minimize unsightly wear and tear. His tan suede ballet-wrap tunic has deconstructionist-style leather top stitching—to conceal unseemly snags. And his studded leather belt/sword holster is wide and snug—to prevent unwelcome hernias. Hand-and-wrist guards with built-in silver bracelets decorate his wrists; brown leather boots protect his feet. Apparently, Rockports haven't made it out to ancient Greece. His cohort, Iolaus, favors black leather pants, and a patchwork woven vest that looks like it hasn't been washed since Homer's return. The Gods of Grunge would be pleased.

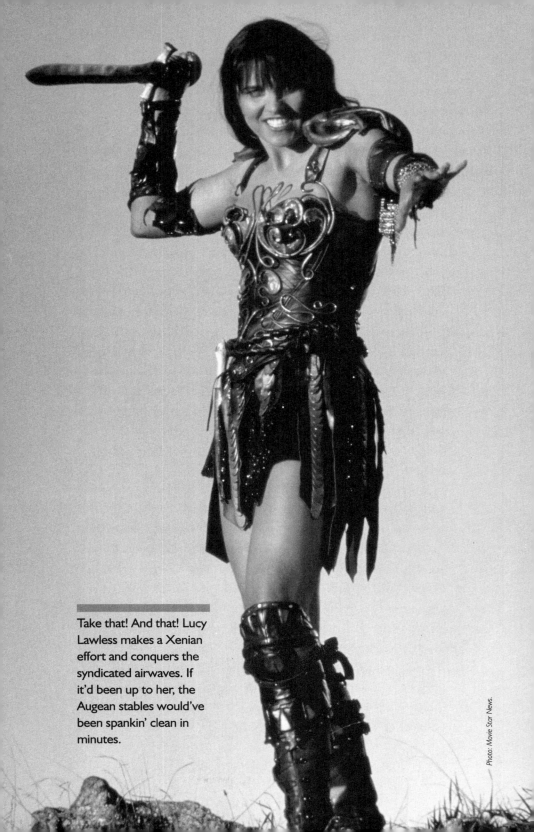

Take that! And that! Lucy Lawless makes a Xenian effort and conquers the syndicated airwaves. If it'd been up to her, the Augean stables would've been spankin' clean in minutes.

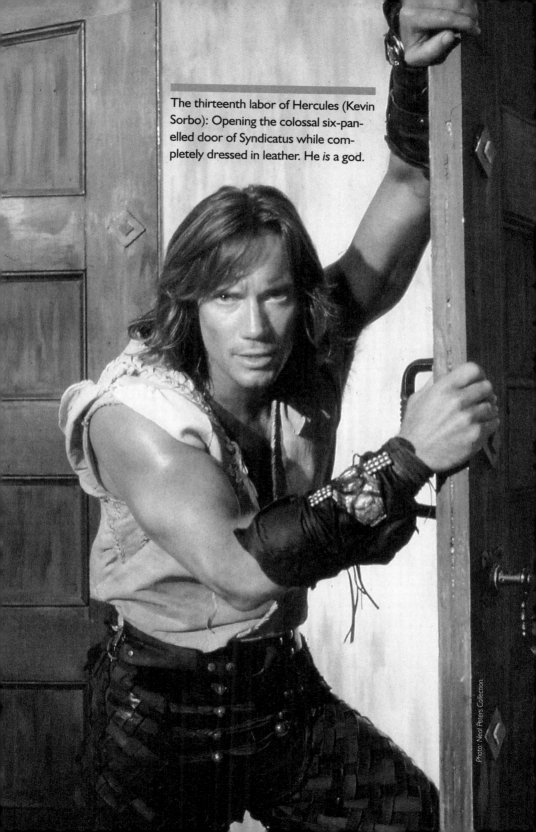

The thirteenth labor of Hercules (Kevin Sorbo): Opening the colossal six-panelled door of Syndicatus while completely dressed in leather. He *is* a god.

Standings: To date, Xena and Hercules have defeated vast armies, Hera, Mars, and other assorted immortals. While Hercules's place in the ratings is certainly secure, underdog Xena has been elevated to the most-watched woman in syndicated TV history—even more watched than notorious *Baywatch*ed bunny, Pamela Anderson Lee (or as you might remember her, PAL!).

The Away Team

Team captain: Professor Dick Soloman (John Lithgow).

Roster: Information Officer Tommy Soloman (Joseph Gordon-Levitt); Military Officer Sally Soloman (Kristen Johnson); Cuddly Mascot Harry Soloman (French Stewart).

Uniform: Due to their covert mission to infiltrate and observe earthling behavior, *3rd Rock*'s uniforms are closer to regular clothes—but they're created in concordance with a team philosophy. "We wanted to come up with a romantic time-traveler look for them," says costume designer Melina Root—hence, the Four Aliens in Search of a Workable Style effect. "They should appear subtly wrong," she adds, "as though they're not entirely sure how to dress on Earth." Root's first costuming dilemma: Where did they get their clothes? The answer: a cosmic Salvation Army that carried clothes from every fashion era of the twentieth century.

As such, Dick's rumpled academic wardrobe was inspired by images of tweedy 1930s-era college professors in muted colors. To give him an alien twist, Root threw in old trench coats, a superabundance of patterns, ties that are always too short, and belts with suspenders. "We go for overkill," says Root. "A plaid tie, a plaid shirt, and a plaid coat give the perfect 'more is more' look." Even so, he gets our vote for tenure, any day.

Tommy, the oldest alien in the youngest human body, is

a *3rd Rocker*—or just look like one.

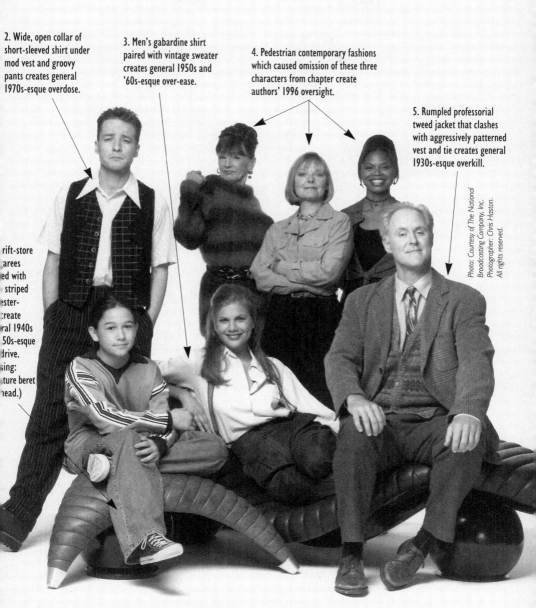

2. Wide, open collar of short-sleeved shirt under mod vest and groovy pants creates general 1970s-esque overdose.

3. Men's gabardine shirt paired with vintage sweater creates general 1950s and '60s-esque over-ease.

4. Pedestrian contemporary fashions which caused omission of these three characters from chapter create authors' 1996 oversight.

5. Rumpled professorial tweed jacket that clashes with aggressively patterned vest and tie creates general 1930s-esque overkill.

rift-store
arees
d with
striped
ester-
create
ral 1940s
50s-esque
drive.
sing:
ture beret
head.)

Clockwise from top left: Harry Soloman (French Stewart), Mrs. Dubcek (Elmarie Wendel), Dr. Mary Albright (Jane Curtin), Nina (Simbi Khali), Dick Soloman (John Lithgow), Sally Soloman (Kristen Johnston), Tommy Soloman (Joseph Gordon-Levitt) reminiscent of the forties and fifties. "We wanted him to have a contemporary, oversized schoolboy silhouette—but in vintage clothing," says Root. She puts him in bowling shirts, used dungarees found in thrift stores, army pants from the World War II era, and old Converse sneakers. Apparently, Rockports have made it out to Ohio—and he doesn't give a tinker's cuss. His colors are primary, and the beret is a permanent fixture—even in real Earth life.

Moving right along to the fifties and sixties, Sally maintains a low-maintenance profile in men's gabardine shirts, old Levi's corduroys, vintage T-shirts, antique sweaters, and lace-up combat boots. Because citizens on her planet have no gender (or body, for that matter), "Sally is constantly at odds with this society's emphasis on women's looks," explains Root. "Her clothes are always too big, too small, too loose, or too tight—I wanted to convey a sense of what real women have to go through when they get dressed on a daily basis." When she gussies up, no holds are barred. "She doesn't understand the concept of being appropriately dressed," says Root. "She swings from one extreme to the next." In a single episode, for instance, she might go from total tomboy to what Root refers to as "Hot Sally": tight spaghetti strap dresses with yards of leg (Johnson is six feet tall), full hair and makeup, and "the highest heels in America." In space, no one can hear your feet scream.

Finally, Harry dances to a wild and woolly seventies beat, albeit in his own herky-jerky style. "He's obsessed with weird notions of the everyday," says Root. "He'll sit and stroke the couch for hours." As a sort of family pet, Harry wears a huge fur parka, as well as large-collared shirts and oversized pleated pants. He also experiments with strange layering, such as short-sleeved shirts over a long-sleeved T-shirt. Bright colors and contrasting prints put him even more on edge. "Buster

Keaton is my inspiration for Harry," says Root. "I find most of his stuff in costume showrooms and movie studio warehouses." For the rest of the cast, she frequents vintage stores like Iguana and Jet Rag. And like most families, the Solomans are wont to swap clothes. Sally might wear Dick's cardigans, or Harry might borrow one of Sally's shirts (but nobody lays a finger on Tommy's beret). "I want them to look unique, but not so unique that they stick out," says Root. "Ultimately, they want to fit into their surroundings." Don't we all?

Standings: After ABC turned down *3rd Rock*, NBC picked it up—and it became the runaway hit of the 1996 midseason. To add astronomical insult to injury, the dark-horse sitcom then started beating out its competition, ABC's *Roseanne*. For the Big Heads of the networks, it was the thrill of victory, the agony of defeat . . . the sweet nectar of success, the bitter dregs of failure. . . . **The Best of Prime Time, the Worst of Prime Time**. In Trek-speak, that would be **Chapter XIV**.

Chapter Fourteen

The Best of Prime Time, the Worst of Prime Time

P hew. It's been quite a ride, hasn't it? After talking to more than forty experts about nearly two hundred television characters, we've seen the best—and worst—of prime-time style. Our brains have been distressed, altered, tailored, fitted, pleated, hemmed, cuffed, buttoned, overdyed, unzipped, and color-saturated within an inch of their cerebral lives. And now, having reported on everyone and their mother's and their mother's dog's opinions, it's time for us—you know, Val and Ellen—to weigh in. At first, we couldn't decide how to organize our thoughts, but then we figured, what the hell? Why not try something new and exciting like categories? That'll really throw our readers for a loop!

Character We'd Most Want to Dress Like

Without pause, Val picked Valerie (Tiffani-Amber Thiessen) on *90210* for her curvy, sexy, take-no-bullshit style of dressing. Ellen personally thinks that Valerie (the character, not the co-author) is too stuffed into her clothes, and considers her a walking sausage in heels. Val personally likes sausage. In any case, Ellen's choice: Teri Hatcher from *Lois and Clark*, for her elegant, clean, timeless aesthetic. Granted, she's sleeping with a guy who wears tights. We're willing to overlook this for the sake of our craft.

Character We Most Often End Up Dressing Like

Due to Val's predilection for unstructured, Bohemian garments, she compared herself to Brett Butler's Grace (as in *Under Fire*). Ellen would like to emphasize that Val is much, much prettier than Brett Butler, not to mention much younger and much thinner. Val is grateful for Ellen's kind support. On the other hand, Ellen's closet parallels Alison's (Courtney Thorne-Smith) from *Melrose Place* on account of her A-line dresses, short skirts, and heeled loafers. Val would like to emphasize that Ellen is much, much better adjusted than Alison, not to mention much better employed and much more in control of her alcohol intake. Ellen is grateful for Val's kind support, although, quite honestly, she would've preferred words like "prettier," "younger," and "thinner."

Character We'd Most Want Our Boyfriends to Dress Like

Val's fondest wish is for aliens to abduct her boyfriend and return him to earth looking like Fox Mulder from *The X-Files*. He's so dreamy; he makes her dream and dream and dream. She is not alone. While Ellen agrees that David Duchovny is one heck of a handsome man (smart, too!), she'd like her boyfriend to dress like *Friends*'s Chandler

(Matthew Perry), because he's kinda free, kinda now—Chandler; kinda she, kinda wow—Chandler! (There's a drug that she needs today, and they call it Valium!)

Character Our Boyfriends Most Often End Up Dressing Like

Fashion-wise, Val's main squeeze most closely resembles Charlie Salinger (Matthew Fox . . . Mulder?) on *Party of Five*, who is also dreamy but a total slob, and if you don't mind, she'd rather not discuss it anymore, okay? Astonishingly, Ellen's best boy does dress exactly like Chandler! *Quelle* fluke. It's like she planned it, or something. *Or something.*

Character Whose Hair We'd Most Like to Have

Val went with Jane Leeves on *Frasier* because Daphne's hair is everything her own hair isn't: straight, shiny, smooth, thick, and seemingly unaffected by humidity. At this juncture, Ellen would like to point out that if Val weren't so lazy in the morning and actually made the effort to, uh, blow-dry, her hair *could* look just like Daphne's. Val maintains that it's not the blow dryer she has a problem with, it's that confusing big, round brush. Ellen's best-tressed vote went to Josie Bissett on *Melrose Place*, because Jane's hair is everything her own hair isn't: short, pixie-ish, and blond as a fresh, new butter pat. At this juncture, Val would like to point out that if Ellen weren't so Asian in the morning, her hair could look just like Jane's. Ellen maintains there's nothing she can do about it.

Character Whose Hair We Really Do Have

Val's hair could pass as Darlene Connor's hair (Sara Gilbert on *Roseanne*). And Ellen's hair is a dead ringer for . . . well, gee, let's see, let's think, hmmm, hmmm, that would be, gosh, out of the hundreds of characters on TV, whose could

Ellen's hair look like? Only one: Trudy (Ming-Na Wen) on *The Single Guy*. Funny how that works.

Characters We Most Admire for Pulling It Off, Despite Their Fashion Disadvantages

Val asserts that Xena (Lucy Lawless) does a terrific job of not looking like a major boob in her breastplate and straps. In the same superhuman vein, Ellen admires Superman (Dean Cain) for his ability to be debonair in a cape and unitard with a huge logo emblazoned on the front. Logos are *so* tacky.

Characters We're Most Appalled by for Not Being Able to Pull It Off, Despite Their Fashion Advantages

Donna (Tori Spelling) on *90210*. Got an hour?

Character We'd Most Like to Stare Up at from the Operating Table

While Ellen and Val are both mesmerized by the feral bedside eyes and devil-may-care wardrobe of *Chicago Hope*'s Dr. Billy Kronk (Peter Berg), Val also has a weakness for Frasier Crane's (Kelsey Grammer) vested finesse. Unfortunately, if Frasier were operating on her, it'd probably be for a lobotomy, in which case clothing would be kind of irrelevant.

Character We'd Most Like to Operate On

Amanda (Heather Locklear) on *Melrose Place* gave Val the urge to renovate; she's dying to snap Amanda out of her oxygen-depriving suits and show off her natural beauty with jeans and T-shirts. Ellen agreed, but had a bigger hankering to overhaul Corky (Faith Ford) on *Murphy Brown*. Frankly, wrapping a body like that in Ann Taylor is a shocking waste of natural resources. Just because you admire Hillary Rodham Clinton doesn't mean you should dress like her.

Character We'd Most Like to Start a Trend

Val chose Ellen—and this flattered Ellen immensely until she realized that Val really meant Ellen DeGeneres, at which point she stormed out in a huff. The reason: Val's been wearing Vans for years, and is happy to see someone on TV picking up the tread. She also would like DeGeneres's relaxed, smart trouser style to catch on, and finds comfort in the fact that someone on TV wears a size eight. When she came back from her huff, Ellen (the co-author, not the character) opted for Carey Lowell on *Law & Order* due to her quintessential, basic-black Calvin Kleinishness. After several seasons of blue, brown, green, and gray being hailed as the "new black," Ellen fervently hopes that true black will make a comeback. Hey, that rhymes!

Character Whose Trend We'd Most Like to Forget Besides Rachel's Haircut

If Val never sees another pair of low-slung, midriff-baring vinyl hip-huggers for the rest of her life (think Kathleen Robertson's Claire of *90210*), it'll be too soon. As for Ellen, those *Clueless* girls' teeny-tiny, little shiny, eensy-weensy backpacks perched in the center of their backs like baby opossums riding home with Momma make her want to . . . to . . . well, to do something really bad, that's what! Bad backpacks! No! Wrong!

Whooo-wee! Glad we got that off our chests. Thanks for joining us on our shopping expedition through *Prime-Time Style*. Hope you learned as much as we did (TV IS EVIL! DON'T BE FOOLED—THOSE ELEC-TRONIC WAVES ARE CONTROLLING YOUR MIND!). And this concludes our broadcast day. Maestro, "The Star-Spangled Banner," please. Beeeeeeeeeeeeeeeeeeeeeeeeeeeeeeeeeep.

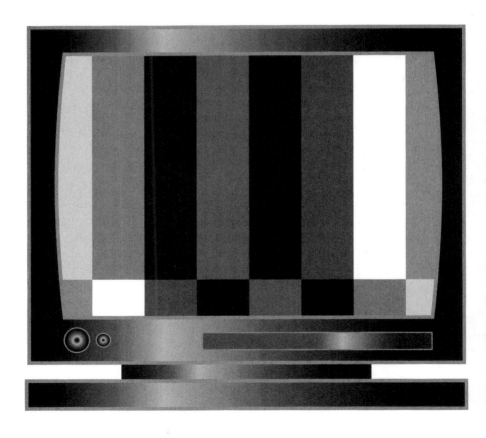